New $14.95

Natural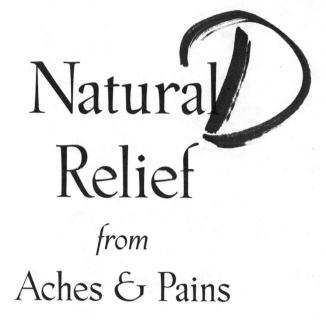
Relief
from
Aches & Pains

Also by CJ Puotinen:

The Encyclopedia of Natural Pet Care

Herbal Teas

Herbs for Detoxification

Herbs for the Heart

Herbs to Help You Breathe Freely

Herbs for Improved Digestion

Herbs for Men's Health

Herbs to Relieve Arthritis

Natural Remedies for Dogs and Cats

Nature's Antiseptics

Natural

Relief

from

Aches & Pains

CJ Puotinen

KEATS PUBLISHING

LOS ANGELES

The purpose of this book is to educate. It is sold with the understanding that the publisher and author shall have neither liability nor responsibility for any injury caused or alleged to be caused by the information contained in this book. While every effort has been made to ensure its accuracy, the book's contents should not be construed as medical advice. Each person's health needs are unique. To obtain recommendations appropriate to your particular situation, please consult a qualified health care provider.

Library of Congress Cataloging-in-Publication Data
Puotinen, CJ,
    Natural relief from aches & pains / CJ Puotinen
      p.   cm.
    Includes bibliographical information and index.
    ISBN 0-658-01146-4 (paper)
      1. Naturopathy. 2. Medicine, Popular. I. Title: Natural relief from
      aches & pains
    RZ440.P86 2001
    615.5'35—dc21

                                    00-065541

Published by Keats Publishing
4255 West Touhy Avenue
Lincolnwood (Chicago), Illinois 60712-1975 U.S.A.

Interior design by Robert S. Tinnon
This book was set in Bembo by Robert S. Tinnon Design
Printed and bound by R.R. Donnelley & Sons

International Standard Book Number: 0-658-01146-4

00 01 02 03 04 05 DOH/DOH 18 17 16 15 14 13 12 11 10 9 8 7 6 5 4 3 2 1

Contents

Contents

Acknowledgments

As always, I am indebted to those who have shared their knowledge and expertise. My teacher, Rosemary Gladstar, continues to inspire herbalists everywhere with her wisdom, discoveries, common sense, and love of life. Dora Gerber, who let me work as an apprentice at her Swissette Herb Farm in Salisbury Mills, New York, introduced me to the healing traditions of Western Europe. Jean Argus, founder of Jean's Greens Herbal Tea Works, is as generous with information as she is a meticulous and accomplished herbalist. Suzanne Catty and Kristen Leigh Bell showed me the fascinating world of therapeutic-quality essential oils and hydrosols, a large step beyond popular aromatherapy. David Winston, James Green, and other leading herbalists have always been generous with their time and knowledge. For a better understanding of human nutrition, I am indebted to the anthropologists, nutritionists, and researchers described in chapters 2 and 3. Claudia McCowan, my editor at Keats and NTC/Contemporary Publishing, suggested this book, which includes portions of three of my books from the Keats Good Herb Guide series: *Herbs for Improved Digestion, Herbs to Help You Breathe Freely,* and *Herbs to Relieve Arthritis.* To all, my gratitude and appreciation.

Introduction

INDIGESTION, ULCERS, HAY FEVER, asthma, bronchitis, gout, colds, flu, arthritis, fibromyalgia, muscle strains, headaches, and assorted other aches and pains change the lives and restrict the activities of millions of Americans every day.

These discomforts can be mildly annoying or life-threatening, and a good part of modern medicine is devoted to treating their symptoms.

Masking symptoms with drugs may bring temporary improvement, but this approach seldom cures a chronic illness. Over time, most prescription drugs lose their effectiveness, requiring larger doses or changes to stronger medication. In conventional Western medicine, chronic diseases can't be cured, prevented, or reversed; instead, they are "managed" by suppressing their symptoms for as long as possible.

Natural therapies are growing in popularity for several reasons. In addition to costing less, they often work as well as or better than their orthodox counterparts. They seldom have adverse side effects and are supported by decades or centuries of use. Most importantly, they help place control over one's body and destiny where it rightly belongs, at home with the individual and her family.

There are basically two ways to use alternative therapies. The first and more common, at least in the United States, is to seek a natural product that will alleviate symptoms the way a prescription drug might but with less risk and expense. This thinking has made fractionated nutritional supplements, standardized herbal extracts, and clinically tested products a billion-dollar industry.

Although this approach is often called holistic, it isn't, for it doesn't attempt to treat the whole person. Like conventional Western medicine, it focuses on inflamed joints, stomach pains, and other specific symptoms. Symptom-oriented medicine examines whatever part of the body is most affected, then seeks a drug or procedure that will counteract the conditions affecting that part. Holistic medicine takes a different approach. Instead of focusing on specific symptoms, holistic medicine examines the whole patient in an effort to determine which diet, exercise, and lifestyle changes will bring the body into balance and stimulate healing from within.

This book takes both approaches, offering simple therapies that temporarily relieve symptoms while focusing on the nutritional and lifestyle changes that are most likely to effect lasting cures. There is no single treatment for any condition, and no therapy works for everyone, but the following treatments work well for people around the world of all ages, races, and backgrounds to relieve pain and discomfort.

Please note: If you are now taking prescription drugs for relief from the symptoms of a chronic condition or if you suffer from a serious illness, it is important to work with an experienced health care practitioner before experimenting with alternative therapies. In the Resources, you will find organizations, books, magazines, newsletters, and other sources of information. These listings and the professional directories of alternative health care services available in many health food stores and libraries can help you locate a qualified practitioner in your area.

While living in a tropical climate in my twenties, I experimented with fasting and vegetarianism. New York's colder climate took me back to an omnivorous diet, but soon I was experimenting with macrobiotics, then the Pritikin diet, and finally a grain-based vegetarian diet. For four of the last fifteen years I was a strict vegan and consumed no animal products. For most of one year I ate only raw food, and for a month during that year I was a fruitarian, eating only raw fruit. Fresh, raw, and organic were my mottos. I went on juice fasts, followed herbal detoxification programs, studied the rules of food combining, and monitored my body's acid/alkaline balance with daily pH tests.

When my husband, friends, physicians, and well-intentioned strangers argued that some people need meat, everyone needs fat, and what I really needed was a good steak, I knew they were uninformed and misguided. All Americans, I knew, would be healthy if only they adopted a low-fat, cholesterol-free, meat-free diet.

Well, what I didn't know could fill a book, and here it is. I've learned to appreciate the wisdom of traditional diets from around the world and the very different ways in which foods react with individual body chemistries. I'm not ready for steak, but I'm no longer a vegan, and I no longer assume that I know which diet is best for anyone else.

I hope you will find practical information and useful resources here and that when you try them, these methods will help you enjoy a more active, pain-free, and enjoyable life. Please remember that the purpose of this book is not to diagnose any illness or prescribe a specific treatment. Rather, it describes a number of simple, successful therapies and the resources that can inform you about them. Armed with practical knowledge, you can make informed decisions about your own and your family's health and care.

In any book that describes the use of medicinal plants, their correct identification is essential. Introducing an herb with both its common name and Latin name avoids confusion but makes sentences unwieldy, especially when several plants are mentioned together. I tried to strike a balance by using the full names of popular herbs whose Latin names typically appear on product labels, and those of plants used to make therapeutic-quality essential oils, or whenever warranted. For more detailed information about any plant mentioned here, see the Resources and Bibliography at the end of this book.

Readers are invited to send comments to the author at the address below. For a personal reply, please enclose a self-addressed, stamped envelope.

CJ PUOTINEN
P.O. Box 525
Hoboken, NJ 07030-0525

Natural Relief

from

Aches & Pains

CHAPTER ONE

Simple, Holistic Ways to Improve Your Health

THE FOLLOWING CHAPTERS describe several ways to treat conditions that cause discomfort, such as digestive disorders, respiratory problems, arthritis, and injuries.

Because these treatments do not involve drugs or surgery, they are called holistic. Holistic therapy involves the whole being, not just its parts, and the single treatment that best addresses the whole being is nutrition. With the right fuel, the body functions perfectly; without it, all kinds of things go wrong. As soon as the right nutrients are provided in the correct proportions, the body begins to repair itself. The repair may take time, especially in conditions that took years to develop, but with continued optimum nutrition, the good results can be permanent. Nothing in holistic health care is as important as discovering and providing the best diet for your unique body chemistry.

There is an unfortunate tendency among nutritionists and physicians to assume that all human beings are identical and that once the "best" diet is discovered, everyone will thrive on it. But people aren't identical, and the foods that keep your best friend in perfect health may make you ill, and vice versa. Fascinating discoveries about nutrition and health are being made every day, and they deserve our attention. Chapters 2 and 3 will help you discover which foods provide the nutrition your body chemistry requires.

In addition to eating the right foods, there are several things you can do to improve your health in a general way. These suggestions apply to everyone, regardless of symptoms. All too often, natural therapies such as herbs, essential oils, and nutritional supplements are used as replacements for conventional medical treatments. Yes, they have fewer side effects than prescription drugs, but if you have a symptom and look only for an herb that will make it go away, you're thinking like an orthodox physician. Choosing an herb, essential oil, nutritional supplement, or other natural products as a direct replacement for a prescription drug is just as shortsighted as the conventional therapy it replaces. At their best, natural therapies do far more than provide temporary relief from pain and discomfort; they effect permanent cures. But they are most likely to accomplish the latter when combined with general rather than symptom-specific treatments that stimulate healing from within.

Whatever your condition, the following suggestions will help you attain and maintain optimum health.

EAT SOMETHING RAW

In the 1930s, the French chemist Paul Kouchakoff discovered that as soon as cooked or processed food is tasted, white blood cells rush to the intestines. This phenomenon, called digestive leucocytosis, disrupts the immune system; the body regards cooked food as a pathogen and works hard to destroy it. Kouchakoff found that the more processed or refined the food, the stronger the reaction. Over time, this energy-consuming emergency response weakens the system.

When Kouchakoff's volunteers ate only raw food, their white blood cells remained in place. The same thing happened when they ate something cooked after eating something raw. The body's white blood cells respond to the first bite of food, not the second.

If your first taste of food, before you eat or drink anything else, is raw rather than cooked, you will avoid leucocytosis, improve your digestion, and help strengthen your immune system.

TASTE SOMETHING BITTER

Our tongues have only four kinds of taste buds; they detect sweet, sour, bitter, and salty flavors. In modern America, our sweet and salty taste buds see most of the action, for we are culturally conditioned to avoid sour and bitter tastes. In Europe and other parts of the world, bitters are alive and well, and all of us would benefit from a greater exposure to their pungency. As soon as taste buds detect something bitter, they stimulate the secretion of gastric juices, such as bile from the liver. In addition, bitters have a tonic action on the entire body.

Bitters that improve digestion can be classified into three categories: tonic, aromatic, and hot. Tonic bitters, like gentian root and blessed thistle, are the sharpest tasting and have an immediate effect on the digestive process. Aromatic bitters, like angelica root, myrrh gum, and peppermint, are more fragrant and contain volatile oils. Hot bitters, like gingerroot and horseradish, stimulate circulation in the stomach, intestines, sinuses, and throughout the body.

The late Austrian herbalist Maria Treben made Swedish Bitters a household name in Europe after she discovered its recipe in an old manuscript. Treben documented a hundred effective uses for this tincture (alcohol extract), which she credited with saving her life.

Swedish Bitters is sold in health food stores or you can make your own at home using packaged herbs (see Resources). For improved digestion, take 1 teaspoon diluted with water or straight from the spoon shortly before breakfast and dinner. For best results, hold the bitters on your tongue for half a minute or more before swallowing. For indigestion after eating, take up to 3 tablespoons straight or diluted with water, as needed. For serious ailments, dilute 1 tablespoon in ½ cup herb tea and take half of this before eating and the other half after, repeating the treatment with every meal.

TAKE YOUR TIME

In recent years, the French have fascinated researchers with their unusually low incidence of heart disease despite a diet high in cholesterol, fat, and animal-source protein. Much attention has been paid to the protective benefits of the red wine consumed at most French meals, but a more significant factor is time. The typical French lunch is a low-stress affair that lasts for two hours; dinners are just as relaxed.

Americans, on the other hand, are notorious for eating on the run, swallowing food without tasting it, and eating in stressful surroundings. By taking a lesson from the French, we can improve our digestion, lower high blood pressure, and relieve or prevent many chronic conditions. Eat as slowly as possible in a relaxing environment, take the time to chew your food thoroughly, and savor each bite before swallowing. Avoid arguments at the table, listen to soothing music instead of the news, and turn off cell phones, pagers, computers, and similar distractions. The more demanding and stressful your career, the more important it is to have a stress-free breakfast, lunch, and dinner.

CONSIDER ENZYMES

The heat of cooking and pasteurization destroys enzymes, which are proteinlike catalysts that speed the rate of biological reactions. The most familiar enzymes are associated with digestion, but hundreds of different enzymes stimulate activity throughout the body.

The body produces enzymes, and it utilizes enzymes in the food it digests. However, only raw food contains the enzymes that support its digestion; the heat of cooking and pasteurization destroys enzymes. Digestive enzymes taken with meals help digest food, and the same enzymes taken between meals help remove partially digested fats and proteins from the bloodstream and other parts of the body. This strategy, called systemic oral enzyme therapy, is widely used in Europe to treat and prevent chronic illnesses and to speed recovery from injuries. See pages 91 to 92.

DRINK MORE WATER

Perhaps the simplest therapy recommended for chronic health problems is water. In his book *Your Body's Many Cries for Water*, F. Batmanghelidj, M.D., explains that most illness is caused not by pathogens or immune disorders, but by dehydration. "You're not sick," he declares, "you're thirsty." Plain drinking water consumed in sufficient quantity throughout the day helps prevent many medical problems.

Dehydration, even partial or mild dehydration, has been linked by mainstream physicians as well as by Dr. Batmanghelidj with many conditions that cause discomfort, including colitis, dyspepsia, hiatial hernia, osteoarthritis, rheumatoid arthritis, low back pain, neck pain, angina, headaches, stress, depression, high blood pressure and cholesterol, excess body weight, asthma, allergies, diabetes, insomnia, vertigo, cancer (especially colon, breast, and urinary tract cancers), kidney stones, diminished coordination, short-term memory loss, constipation, and an increased probability of adverse side effects from over-the-counter and prescription drugs. Some health care practitioners report that a surprising number of older patients with symptoms of dementia recover as soon as they consume sufficient water.

Dr. Batmanghelidj cautions that fluids like coffee and cola don't count; plain, room-temperature water, up to a gallon a day with a pinch of salt added, brings best results. Most nutritionists and health experts recommend a minimum of eight 8-ounce cups (64 ounces, or 2 quarts) of drinking water daily, and those who are pregnant or nursing, on a high-fiber diet, living at a high altitude or in a hot or dry climate, traveling long distances, especially by air, dieting to lose weight, recovering from an illness, walking or hiking long distances, or participating in athletic events should drink more.

No discussion of water would be complete without a caution regarding American tap water, which has received much negative publicity in recent years. According to a study published in the July 1992 *American Journal of Public Health,* trihalomethanes in chlorinated drinking water are likely responsible for an estimated 4,200 cases of bladder cancer and 6,500 cases of rectal cancer every year. Other studies have linked chlorine to heart disease and other illnesses. Fluoride, which is added to most municipal water supplies, has been linked to brittle bones in the elderly. Industrial chemicals, pesticides, prescription drug residues, contamination from agricultural runoff, and microscopic parasites add additional risks, especially because several organisms have become resistant to chlorine. Public health officials warn that chlorine water treatment plants should be replaced with other technologies, but the conversion will take decades.

In the meantime, concerns over water safety have made bottled spring water a growth industry along with home water filters and distillers. Whatever you can do to improve the quality of the water you drink and bathe in will improve your health.

RECONSIDER SALT

Americans are so used to hearing physicians' warnings against salt that Dr. Batmanghelidj's advice to add a pinch of salt to drinking water sounds strange at first. Refined table salt is associated with high blood pressure, but only a tiny fraction of patients with hypertension have been shown to benefit from a salt-free diet. In contrast to American physicians, who for decades considered low blood pressure an unqualified virtue, European physicians have long regarded hypotension (low blood pressure) a medical condition as potentially harmful as hypertension (high blood pressure).

In 1997, the *Journal of the American Medical Association* published research showing that the salt-free diets recommended for patients with high blood pressure for nearly a century have no therapeutic benefits. Only 2 to 5 percent of patients who followed a salt-free diet experienced any reduction of blood pressure, and that was so slight (only three to five points), it was insignificant. Over 95 percent of the salt-free patients in all the studies conducted over ninety-five years showed no benefit at all.

In fact, avoiding salt causes significant harm to the body. No-salt diets have been shown to contribute to heart disease, chronic fatigue syndrome, and other medical problems. Electrolytes are electricity-conducting ions such as sodium, potassium, and chloride, which circulate in the blood. Electrolyte imbalances disrupt the nervous system and lead to muscle weakness throughout the body, including the heart. Blood pressure that drops when a person stands after lying down, called a positive Ragland test sign, is usually caused by insufficient electrolytes and depleted adrenal glands. No-salt diets have also been shown to cause chronic indigestion. Without adequate salt, the stomach is unable to produce the enzymes and acids needed for efficient digestion, which leads to vitamin deficiencies and other problems caused by the malabsorption of nutrients.

Salt-free diets and chemical salt substitutes harm the body, but so does most of the salt in our food supply. Refined table salt has two main sources, salt mines and ocean flats. Salt company profits come from sales to industry, which requires pure chemicals such as sodium chloride and magnesium for manufacturing. Table salt production constitutes a small portion, about 7 percent, of the business. Trace minerals are refined out of table salt not because they are impurities but because they are too valuable to waste on retail customers.

All popular brands of table salt have been bleached, then treated with stabilizing agents and dehydrating chemicals. Whether coarse or finely ground, this salt is between 98 and 99 percent pure sodium chloride (NaCl). High-temperature drying, nutrient stripping, and added chemicals make table salt difficult for the body to assimilate, contributing to electrolyte imbalances, trace mineral deficiencies, and digestive problems. The sodium content of nearly every processed food derives from refined salt.

Most sea salt is as processed as table salt and contains added chemicals as well. A large French company extracts sea salt by bulldozer from concrete beds along the Mediterranean coast, a seriously polluted area, then refines and sells it as "natural sea salt." Most Mexican sea salt is dried outdoors over an extended period, during which rainstorms leach away desirable minerals. Many brands of sea salt are treated with undisclosed chemicals and most are kiln-dried or boiled. Nearly all are 98 to 99 percent pure sodium chloride and, like table salt, contain no trace minerals, only the residue of processing chemicals.

Fortunately, traditionally harvested unrefined sea salt is imported from France and other countries; three superior brands are Celtic, Eden, and Lima, all of which are sold in health food stores and some markets (see Resources). Natural salt is of special interest to herbalists, for traditionally herbal teas were served salted to enhance their healing properties. A pinch of unrefined salt added to a glass of water or a pot of tea helps balance the body's electrolytes and provides trace minerals often lacking in the food we eat. This salt is also of interest to cooks, for its interaction with food is noticeably different from that of refined table salt. Fermented foods, such as sauerkraut, unpasteurized dill pickles made without vinegar, sourdough bread, and lactic-acid fermented vegetables are all improved by the use of unrefined salt. Because the heat of cooking destroys the more fragile trace elements in unrefined salt, it is best added to food just before serving.

AVOID SUGAR

In nutritional circles, no one has anything good to say about white sugar and only a few defend honey, brown rice syrup, barley malt, maple syrup, dehydrated sugar cane juice, or molasses. Some condemn dried fruit and bottled fruit juices, and a few say we should avoid any fresh fruit sweeter than a cranberry.

This is difficult advice for Americans, whose sweet tooth is rivaled only by that of the English. To maintain our impressive national consumption of refined white sugar, many of us eat half a pound or more per day. Processed foods often contain hidden sugars, such as maltose, dextrose, fructose, and glucose. Add corn syrup, which is the cheapest sweetener available, and it's no wonder our bodies are stressed.

Sugar disrupts digestion by overworking the pancreas, which produces insulin, the hormone that regulates our utilization of glucose and carbohydrates. Excessive insulin, especially in overweight people, is associated with fluid retention, sleep disorders, the production of the "bad" cholesterol (LDL), low metabolism, thyroid disorders, hypoglycemia, and food cravings. Sugar disrupts the immune system and temporarily lowers immunity, which makes it a dangerous food choice when colds, the flu, and other infectious diseases are going around. Internal parasites love sugar. So does *Candida albicans,* the organism that causes chronic yeast infections.

High-fructose corn syrup is of growing concern because large quantities of high-fructose sweeteners can lead to chromium deficiency, which is associated with heart disease and diabetes. In animal studies, overconsumption of high-fructose sweeteners has produced anemia, cardiovascular risk factors, and abnormalities of the heart and pancreas.

Sugar is addictive, and in our culture it is difficult to avoid, but reducing or eliminating sugar from the diet improves digestion, increases energy, and improves overall health.

AVOID ARTIFICIAL SWEETENERS

Americans spend billions of dollars annually on artificial sweeteners. By far the most widely used chemical sweetener is aspartame, the active ingredient in NutraSweet and many processed foods. The U.S. Food and Drug Administration refused to approve aspartame, which its researchers considered dangerous and unstable, until key political appointments changed the product's fortunes. Mary Nash Stoddard, founder of the Aspartame Consumer Safety Network (see Resources), has documented aspartame's colorful history. Stoddard notes that the majority of non-drug complaints to the FDA regard adverse reactions to aspartame; currently, the rate is about 78 percent of all complaints logged, but it has been as high as 85 percent. None of these consumer complaints or information about aspartame-related deaths have been reported in the media. Aspartame causes individual symptoms, including grand mal seizures, and can mimic entire symptoms, such as chronic fatigue and immune deficiency syndromes. According to the medical experts Stoddard interviewed, such as H. J. Roberts, M.D., aspartame can cause decreased vision, eye pain, decreased tears, ringing in the ears, hearing impairment, headache, dizziness, unsteadiness, confusion, memory loss, drowsiness, sleepiness, slurring of speech, numbness, tingling, tremors, depression, irritability, aggression, insomnia, phobias, heart palpitations, shortness of breath, high blood pressure, nausea, diarrhea, abdominal pain, itching, hives, menstrual changes, weight gain, hair thinning, hair loss, urinary burning, urinary frequency, excessive thirst, fluid retention, bloating, increased infection, and in extreme cases death.

By 1998, the Aspartame Consumer Safety Network's Pilot's Hotline had taken over five hundred calls documenting aspartame-related flight safety impairments, including grand mal seizures in the cockpit, vision loss, vertigo, and heart problems. These are symptoms that go far beyond simple headaches, and they are reported by individuals, such as airline and military pilots, who are not usually associated with hypochondria.

Saccharine, America's second most popular artificial sweetener, has far fewer side effects but is blamed for some laboratory animal cancers and has a pronounced chemical flavor.

The herb stevia (*Stevia rebaudiana*), a native of Peru, is widely used as a sugar substitute in Europe, South America, and Asia. Despite its well-documented history of safe use, the FDA does not allow it to be labeled as a sweetener. For a few years, in response to complaints from an artificial sweetener manufacturer the agency refused to name, the FDA banned its importation. The stevia ban has since been lifted, and the herb is sold in health food stores as a liquid extract, bulk herb, and powdered extract. It is an estimated one hundred to three hundred times sweeter than sugar, has no adverse side effects, and is safe for diabetics. Note that some stevia products contain additional ingredients, such as maltodextrin or fructooligosaccharides.

The Indian herb *Gymnema sylvestre* is known in Hindi as *Gumara*, which means "destroyer of sugar." Traditionally used to treat diabetes and sugar cravings, gymnema has two interesting effects. If you taste it, even briefly, it interferes with the taste buds that detect sweetness. A teaspoon of sugar tastes like sand, an effect that lasts up to three hours. At the same time, the herb interferes with sugar receptor sites in the intestines, so that up to 50 percent of ingested sugar passes through the body unabsorbed. Stevia and gymnema products are so popular that most health food stores carry several brands.

See the Resources for a new no-calorie sweetener made from kiwi fruit.

GET THE RIGHT EXERCISE

Two people eat the same foods, drink the same water, live in the same neighborhood, and work in the same office. One enjoys long walks with the family dog and goes dancing several times a week. The other sits at a computer all day and watches TV all night. Guess which one suffers from constipation, stiff joints, fluid retention, depression, and other discomforts?

In addition to eating all the wrong things, Americans are alarmingly under-exercised. An active lifestyle does more than improve circulation and help you lose weight; it improves digestion, elimination, range of motion, skin health, and disposition. Fresh air and aerobic activity are obvious prescriptions for improved health, but did you know that inverted postures are just as important? Yoga offers several upside-down positions, all of which are known for their digestive and rejuvenating benefits, but even reclining at a slight angle on a slant board for five to ten minutes per day has helped many people improve regularity without laxatives, enjoy favorite foods without after-dinner discomfort, sleep more soundly, and improve their appearance. Another beneficial side effect of lying on a slant board, as reported by middle-aged men, is the reversal of prostate symptoms.

One of the least appreciated parts of the body—in Western medicine at least—is the lymph system. Lymph is the clear fluid that contains lymphocytes (the immune system's T-cells and B-cells) and which circulates through lymph channels to filter waste and bacteria from the bloodstream. Lymph circulation improves with active exercise and deep, diaphragmatic breathing. In fact, deep breathing alone can improve lymph circulation. Most Westerners breathe shallowly, filling only the upper portion of the lungs. The slow, deep breathing taught in yoga and meditation classes involves the entire upper body and abdomen. To improve lymph circulation while you breathe, let the stomach relax and inhale slowly, as though you are inflating your abdomen like a balloon. Some instructors suggest different counts, such as inhaling for four seconds, holding the breath for four seconds, and exhaling for eight seconds. Others advise breathing as slowly and fully as possible, contracting the abdomen to push air from the lungs in a complete exhalation, and slowly relaxing the abdomen on the inhalation.

Another lymph-stimulating therapy is daily skin brushing with a dry, vegetable-fiber bath brush (the finest are imported from Japan). Starting at the soles of the feet, work up the legs and trunk to the heart, from the palms of the hands up the arms, then across the back and the abdomen. Maintain a gentle pressure for a few days and increase the pressure as your body becomes used to this daily therapy. Vigorous skin brushing for two to four minutes twice per day helps eliminate lymph mucoid through the bowels.

Rebounding is another way to stimulate lymph circulation and improve digestion. Miniature trampolines became so popular in the 1970s that inferior equipment flooded the market, resulting in injuries and disappointing results, and rebounding fell out of favor. Now superior-quality rebounders (see Resources), which are sufficiently springy to stimulate all the body's systems with even a gentle workout, have spawned a revival of this easy form of exercise. According to Linda Brooks, who has taught reboundology for many years, the fastest and most effective way to improve health is to bounce gently before jumping, and to bounce or jump for a few minutes several times per day. "Jumping in installments," she says, "is more effective than jumping for half an hour in one session."

Brooks has worked with hundreds of clients who used this strategy in combination with an improved diet, and—without the use of prescription drugs or other therapies—their heart disease, diabetes, edema, digestive disorders, multiple sclerosis, arthritis, chronic fatigue syndrome, cancer, and other illnesses disappeared or improved dramatically.

Several yoga postures, especially twisting poses, stimulate lymph circulation. Many massage therapists practice lymph-draining techniques. Some medicinal herbs stimulate the lymph system. There are many ways to increase and improve the body's lymph circulation, and they are all worth pursuing. It is important not to disrupt the flow of lymph by wearing a tight-fitting bra, which interferes with the drainage of lymph glands in the armpit area, or tight jeans, which restrict lymph circulation in the legs. Whatever you can do to stimulate lymph circulation is an important investment in your health and longevity.

Many who suffer from edema or fluid retention, the symptoms of which include swollen fingers and ankles, take prescription diuretics, reduce their intake of water, and eliminate salt from their diets to control it. None of these strategies addresses the cause of fluid retention, which often involves poor lymph circulation. Diuretic drugs do pull fluid from the body, but their effectiveness decreases with long-term use, requiring additional medication; in addition, they disrupt the balance of minerals in the body, put stress on the kidneys, have other potentially adverse side effects, and are a leading cause of dehydration. Ironically, limiting the amount of salt and water in the system contributes to edema, because a water-starved body hoards fluid in its cells.

PREVENT MALILLUMINATION

When photobiologist John Ott pioneered time-lapse photography half a century ago, he discovered that the fluorescent lights under which he grew and photographed plants interfered with their normal development. Whenever electric lights or clear glass replaced or interfered with natural sunlight, buds refused to open, fruit refused to ripen, or plants looked spindly and unhealthy. These observations led him to create the first plastic greenhouse, for plastic allows nearly all of the sun's ultraviolet and full-spectrum rays to pass through.

On a visit to a seawater aquarium in Miami, Ott noticed "black-light" ultraviolet tubes over some of the fish aquarium tanks. He learned that the lights had been installed for decorative purposes, to give the fish an eerie and attractive appearance, but the added light had solved a common health problem in aquarium fish (exophthalmus, or pop-eye), and fin-nipping behaviors had disappeared. The aquarium's curators reported that fish considered too fragile to keep in tanks thrive under black-light ultraviolet, and similar observations have been made about birds, reptiles, and other animals in zoos around the world.

A Miami restaurant featured a similar lighting system, and when Ott interviewed the manager, he learned that the lights had been in place for eighteen years. During that time, the waiters, who had been randomly assigned to the restaurant, maintained perfect health and attendance records and were known for their cheerful dispositions and efficient service.

Ott coined the term *malillumination* to describe the health-damaging effects of light deficiencies he observed in plants, pets, captive animals, and humans, including himself. When he stopped wearing sunglasses and exposed his eyes to unfiltered natural light for several hours a day, his severe arthritis disappeared and X rays showed new bone growth in his hip, which eliminated the need for the hip surgery his physicians had prescribed. Malillumination is now known to contribute to sterility and other fertility problems, depression, hostility, suppressed immune function, hair loss, skin damage, cancer, fatigue, a loss of strength and muscle tone, fragile bones, vision problems, and all types of glandular disorders.

Light enters the eyes not only to facilitate vision but to activate the hypothalamus, which in turn controls the nervous and endocrine systems, which regulate functions throughout the body. The pineal, pituitary, adrenal, thyroid, thymus, and sex glands are all directly or indirectly dependent on the eyes' exposure to natural light. Their health in turn affects body temperature, sleep patterns, growth, the immune system, emotions, fluid balance, energy balance, circulation, blood pressure, breathing, reproduction, and aging. Exposure to natural light is crucial to the health of the hormone and immune systems.

Sunlight activates the synthesis of vitamin D in the body, lowers blood pressure, increases the efficiency of the heart, improves electrocardiogram readings and blood profiles of patients with atherosclerosis, reduces cholesterol, assists in weight loss, effectively treats psoriasis and asthma, kills infectious bacteria, and increases hormone levels.

At the same time, everyone agrees that too much ultraviolet light can be harmful. No one, including John Ott, recommends that people stare directly at the sun or limit their outdoor activities to the middle of the day, when the sun's rays are hottest and brightest. But in recent years, the definition of "too much exposure" has become "any exposure at all," and physicians warn their patients to avoid all sun exposure and wear sunglasses that block 100 percent of the ultraviolet spectrum. The result is an epidemic vitamin D deficiency in addition to all the other symptoms of malillumination.

Exposure to natural light, preferably for several hours per day, is necessary for good health. Whenever possible, partake of this essential nutrient. Natural light is any type of outdoor light, not necessarily direct sunlight. A shady screened porch, the shelter of a large tree, even an open window or doorway with northern exposure gives the body what it needs.

Remember that there is no substitute for natural light, not even fixtures advertised as full-spectrum lights. Although several companies advertise full-spectrum light bulbs or tubes, none of these products exactly duplicates natural light. When outdoor activity isn't possible, consider combining cool white fluorescent tubes or regular incandescent bulbs with a black-light ultraviolet fixture installed near the ceiling. This is the same arrangement that kept Ott's Miami sea creatures and restaurant waiters healthy, and its discovery spawned the full-spectrum lighting industry. For more information, read Ott's book *Health and Light*.

It may seem like an oversimplification to say that most ill-nesses, aches, and pains are caused by nutritional deficiencies, de-hydration, insufficient lymph circulation, and a lack of unfiltered natural light, but those are in fact four leading causes of poor health in America today.

By adopting the right diet, drinking sufficient water, eating natural salt, avoiding sugar, getting the right kind of exercise, and exposing yourself to unfiltered natural light as much as possible, you can improve your health dramatically. This is a truly holistic approach to health, and it is the foundation of the most lasting natural cures.

CHAPTER TWO

Food as Medicine

THE ILLNESSES AMERICANS TAKE for granted—arthritis, cancer, heart disease, diabetes, irritable bowel syndrome, ulcers, indigestion, migraine headaches, tooth infections, gingivitis, chronic fatigue syndrome, fibromyalgia, and a host of others— are modern inventions. They didn't become epidemics until people started eating refined white flour, refined sugar, and the canned and processed foods commonly consumed today.

Anthropologists tell us that humans evolved on a constantly changing diet of whatever nature provided. For millions of years, our prehuman ancestors ate approximately equal quantities of raw plants and raw, low-fat meat. As they developed tools and became more efficient hunters, meat increased to 75 percent of the diet. These hunter-gatherers also ate small quantities of nuts, seeds, and ripe fruits when available. There were no grains or dairy products to be had, and there was no way to store or preserve food. Everything was eaten fresh wherever it was found.

The first significant shift in human diet followed the discovery of fire. Cooking softens the cellulose and fiber in plant foods, toughens the proteins in meats, sterilizes food by killing bacteria and other organisms, and alters taste and texture. It makes some foods easier to digest, but it destroys enzymes and other heat-sensitive nutrients, and it causes chemical reactions that alter the body's reaction to food. Eventually, every culture in the world, including the most primitive tribes, cooked at least some of its foods.

A second significant shift in human diet followed the agricultural revolution, when people domesticated plants and then animals. This made it possible to prevent starvation by setting a surplus aside for future use. Because grains store well, they became a staple food. Many researchers and nutritionists believe that the human digestive tract is still adapting to this dietary shift, which took place ten thousand to twenty thousand years ago.

Even after humans began baking bread and roasting a more stable supply of meat, they consumed most of their food raw or only partly cooked. When grains were ground, they were ground whole, never stripped of their bran to make white rice or flour. Vegetables were eaten raw or lightly cooked; they weren't deep fried, cooked in a pressure cooker, canned, irradiated, or microwaved. Salting (in whole, unprocessed, sea or mined salt), fermentation (making, for example, yogurt, sauerkraut, cheese, wine, beer, or pickles), and drying were the only means of preserving perishable foods beyond the harvest. Sugar as we know it didn't exist, sweets like raw honey were rare treats, and salt was never refined to separate its minerals for sale to industry. No one used pesticides, herbicides, preservatives, chemical additives, artificial flavors, chemical sweeteners, or artificial fats. No one drank pasteurized milk, homogenized milk, pasteurized juice, or carbonated colas. Only in the last one hundred fifty years in the industrial West—especially the last fifty years in North America—have traditional foods been replaced by substances to which human digestive organs were never before exposed. Fifty years of technology in millions of years of digestive evolution is like one second in a twenty-four-hour day. We've been eating modern fare for the blink of an eye.

In the 1930s, Dr. Weston Price, a California dentist, and his wife traveled the world in search of cultures that had little or no contact with the industrial West. The Prices lived with and studied the Swiss in remote Alpine valleys; Gaels on Scotland's Outer Hebridian islands; Inuits (formerly called Eskimos) in Alaska; American Indian tribes in northern, western, and central Canada, the western United States, and Florida; Polynesians and Melanesians in the north and south Pacific; Africans in eastern and central Africa; Aborigines in Australia; Malay tribes on islands north of Australia; the Maori in New Zealand; and descendants of ancient civilizations in Peru. Wherever available, the skeletal remains of ancient people and more immediate ancestors were examined as well.

By 1930, all these cultures had some exposure to modern civilization, and they were beginning to import sugar, white flour, canned foods, and vegetable oils. The Prices were able to find groups living side by side, some who had adopted these convenience foods and others who lived entirely on traditional local fare.

As a dentist, Dr. Price was most interested in dental health, and he kept detailed records and took thousands of photographs. He analyzed the natives' traditional and modern diets for calories, minerals, and vitamins, and he studied the chemical reaction of different foods with saliva and its relationship to dental health. In addition, he described the general health of each subject and interviewed the practitioners who provided medical care.

Although these cultures ate very different foods depending on their location and climate, all depended on animals and vegetables. Only the Swiss and some African tribes consumed dairy products such as milk, cheese, or butter, all of which came from healthy, well-exercised animals. Only a few groups consumed grain as a staple food, such as rye in Switzerland, oats in the Outer Hebrides, millet in Africa, and quinoa in Peru.

The Swiss ate mostly whole rye bread and dairy products; once a week they ate meat and used the bones and scraps in soup. Natives of the Outer Hebrides ate oats, fish, and shellfish, very little milk, and no fruit. Alaskan Inuits ate salmon, seal, caribou, kelp, wild plants, and berries. Their fat consumption was the highest of the groups the Prices studied. North American Indians ate a variety of foods typical of hunter-gatherer tribes, including fish, meat, and plants. In Melanesia, Polynesia, and Hawaii, the native diet consisted of shellfish, fish, fruits, sea vegetables, and land plants. Their consumption of fats was the lowest of the groups studied. In Africa, tribes that herded cattle and goats lived on the milk, meat, and blood of their livestock as well as plants, nuts, and fruit. Africa's agricultural tribes grew sweet potatoes, beans, bananas, millet, and other grains. In Australia and New Zealand, traditional cultures living near the ocean ate fish, shellfish, sea vegetables, land plants, and fruit, while inland tribes ate roots, stems, berries, seeds, and every type of animal, as well as insects, fish, and birds. In the Andes Mountains, natives of southern Peru and Bolivia followed the same diet as their Incan ancestors, eating fish, birds, grains, roots, beans, and seeds.

In every group they studied, the Prices found that those who followed the traditional diet had very few decayed teeth; in fact, most groups were completely free of cavities, and so were the skeletons of their ancestors. Cancer, heart disease, arthritis, and other chronic illnesses were unheard of. They were physically strong, well formed, long-lived, and had perfect dental arches and tooth alignment.

A few miles from each of the traditional tribes lived groups identical in every way except that they had changed their diets, adopting imported flour, sugar, and canned foods. In every case, the contrast was dramatic. Dental health suffered immediately, with such extensive tooth decay that some committed suicide to relieve their pain. Previously unknown illnesses, such as tuberculosis, cancer, arthritis, rheumatoid arthritis, and other chronic diseases, became common. So did reproductive problems including prolonged and difficult labors, infertility, miscarriages, and birth defects. The natives' impressive immunity to contagious diseases disappeared and they became susceptible to infectious viruses and bacteria. Children raised on modern food were physically weak and had crowded teeth, narrow rather than broad faces, poorly contoured dental arches, jaw deformities, rampant tooth decay, and all types of illnesses.

In some cases, individuals returned to their traditional diets and their health improved. Tooth decay stopped, and chronic diseases disappeared. Price interviewed local physicians who recommended a return to traditional villages as a medical treatment. Even patients with tuberculosis, which was progressive and usually fatal to natives on refined food, made full recoveries without Western drugs or medical intervention when they resumed their traditional lifestyle.

Price's book *Nutrition and Physical Degeneration* was for many years required reading in college anthropology courses. Unfortunately, it was never read by medical students. Its comprehensive documentation and dramatic photographs still make for compelling reading.

Other medical researchers and anthropologists have studied traditional cultures of the modern and ancient worlds, and their findings have been similar. Traditional cultures in China, Japan, Tibet, the Middle East, South America, the Philippines, Scandinavia, the Caribbean, the Mediterranean, and other parts of the world ate a wide-ranging diet of whole foods.

In the industrial West, few of us understand what whole foods are. We may appreciate that brown rice and whole wheat are whole foods because they contain everything in the natural grain, as opposed to white rice and white flour, which have been stripped of nutrients. We tend to think of bran, a by-product of the milling process that strips those nutrients, as a whole food because it is sold in health food stores. In fact, wheat bran, rice bran, and oat bran are only partial foods. They contain nutrients not found in white flour, white rice, or instant oatmeal, but they are not the same as whole wheat, brown rice, or whole oats. Enriched white bread is not a whole food, either; it contains a few synthetic vitamins that are supposed to compensate for the hundreds of nutrients that are removed before the bread is baked.

Juices are partial foods because they have been separated from the whole fruits and vegetables that were used to make them. Most of the juices sold in supermarkets are even further removed from whole produce because they are diluted with water, sweetened with high-fructose corn syrup, colored with food dyes, and preserved with chemicals. Skim milk and butter are partial foods because they have been separated from the whole milk that came from the cow, and the pasteurized, homogenized product sold as "whole milk" is nothing a calf would recognize. Soy milk and tofu are partial foods because they have been separated from the soybeans used to make them.

In addition to eating whole fruits, whole vegetables, and whole grains, people living in traditional cultures ate whole animals, not skinless and boneless chicken breasts, beef muscle meat, and fish fillets. Organ meats such as the liver, kidneys, spleen, stomach, and eyes; glands such as the thyroid; bones and their marrow, and other animal parts prevented deficiencies and provided vital nutrients.

Of the world's traditional cultures, only the Hindus of India developed a vegetarian diet. This occurred in a warm rather than cold climate, and although their diet did not feature animal flesh, it was not a vegan diet, which is free of all animal products. The Hindu cuisine made (and continues to make) extensive use of cow's milk and butter.

Despite their differences, the diets of traditional cultures studied by Weston Price and others had certain things in common. They consisted of fresh foods that were grown or gathered locally and in season on a planet that was free of industrial chemicals. If preserved, these foods were dried, fermented, pickled, smoked, or salted, all of which are natural methods. The foods were used whole, not refined, and they were often eaten literally whole, not minced, ground, or shredded. Most foods, including many animal foods, were eaten raw. When cooked, foods were heated over an open fire or boiled, steamed, or baked. Grains and legumes were soaked for several hours before cooking.

By adapting these principles to our own menu planning, we can improve our health. For example, it makes sense to use organically grown foods whenever possible. The U.S. Department of Agriculture (USDA) recently announced that the nutritional content of conventionally grown fruits and vegetables declined significantly in the twentieth century. While USDA officials say they cannot account for the change, other researchers have shown that commercial farming practices, including the use of chemical fertilizers that contain only a few nutrients, monoculture (growing a single plant species instead of several), and harvesting methods that do not return organic material to the soil have so depleted the nutrients in America's farmland that everything grown in it is deficient in both vitamins and minerals.

As this book goes to press, there is much confusion about the labeling of organic produce because the USDA is defining national standards that will replace those developed by California, Oregon, and other states. The organic label used to guarantee that produce was grown without the use of chemical fertilizers, sewage sludge, pesticides, fungicides, and other chemicals, using organically produced seeds that were not genetically altered, and that the resulting food was never fumigated or irradiated. Dairy products, eggs, poultry, and meat labeled organic came from animals fed a natural diet without the addition of antibiotics, growth hormones, or rendered animal parts; this last, which is common in factory farming, refers to using the remains of diseased animals as a source of protein in animal feed. Whether the USDA's standard will restrict or allow these questionable practices remains to be seen, but wherever it is mentioned in this book, the term *organic* refers to the standards described above.

Free-range animals, unlike animals raised in factory farms, have access to fresh air, sunlight, and outdoor exercise. Superior-quality organically grown produce and free-range meat and poultry are the first choices of many gourmet chefs, who consider the taste and quality unsurpassed, and who are aware that the abundance of nutrients and absence of toxic residues, including pesticides in produce and antibiotics in meat, poultry, and eggs, provide complete nutrition without stressing the body with contaminants.

Although the best organic produce is grown in land that has been strengthened by the addition of mineral-rich soil amendments such as seaweed, or cover crops that pull minerals from deep in the soil before being tilled back into it, some organic fruits and vegetables are grown in depleted soil and lack the same nutrients as commercially grown crops. However, most health food stores, natural food markets, cooperatives (co-ops), and farmer's markets sell produce grown locally by farmers who work hard to improve the nutritional content of their crops. Talk with produce buyers to discover which crops come from the best local growers. Ask whether anyone in your area uses biodynamic farming practices, which are a step beyond organic. In addition to finding local suppliers, consider growing vegetables in your own or a neighbor's yard or in a community garden. With the help of *Organic Gardening* magazine, library books, adult-school classes, and demonstrations of organic gardening techniques, you can improve your garden every year with a minimum of effort.

In menu planning, use fresh ingredients and whole foods as much as possible. White rice, refined white flour, any type of added sugar, and refined salt should be avoided, along with anything containing chemical preservatives, artificial colors, chemical flavor enhancers, or artificial flavors. This step is difficult because it requires avoiding nearly everything sold in America's supermarkets and restaurants, but chronic disorders such as arthritis, asthma, allergies, and digestive problems can improve rapidly if these strategies are combined with the right diet.

FINDING THE RIGHT DIET

Few subjects excite passionate debate the way food does. Everyone has a favorite way of eating, a favorite diet, a favorite expert, and a favorite nutritional horror story.

The Standard American Diet

According to the U.S. Department of Agriculture and groups like the American Medical Association, the Arthritis Foundation, and the American Heart Association, it's easy to follow a healthful diet. Just eat a balanced variety of foods every day.

These organizations used to endorse the four food groups, which consist of meat, dairy products, breads or grains, and fruits or vegetables. For decades, everyone was encouraged to eat at least one food from each of these categories at every meal. Despite their almost universal endorsement by the medical establishment, the four food groups were not created by food scientists; they were devised as a promotional tool by the meat and dairy industries, which supplied guidelines, sample menus, and educational materials to schools, hospitals, physicians, and the media.

The four food groups eventually fell out of favor and, after much debate, nutritionists endorsed a food pyramid. According to the pyramid, we should make most of our selections from the bottom tier (bread, cereal, rice, and pasta) and the one just above it (vegetables and fruits), while eating substantially less meat, poultry, nuts, dry beans, fish, and dairy products (grouped together because they are protein foods), and only sparing amounts of foods at the pyramid's top, which are fats, oils, and sweets.

While the food pyramid was under construction, meat and dairy groups lobbied for larger portions of meat and dairy products, while vegetarians tried to keep meat out altogether. Researchers, nutritionists, and health care professionals disagreed about the proportions of protein, carbohydrates, and fats a healthy diet should provide. Some favored the 40-30-30 plan, in which 40 percent of every meal consists of carbohydrates,

30 percent is protein, and 30 percent is fat, while others argued for more or less of each component.

So many experts frown on fat that today's marketplace is full of fat-free, cholesterol-free, and "guilt-free" foods. But despite our growing consumption of low-fat and no-fat foods, Americans are fatter than ever. In May 2000, at the first national nutrition summit in thirty-one years, government officials announced that 55 percent of Americans are overweight—more than twice the percentage in 1969—and one out of every four adults is obese.

One reason for the nation's epidemic weight gain is an increased consumption of carbohydrates, especially sugar and white flour. Even snacks made with whole wheat (a "health" food) and fruit juice (a "no-sugar" sweetener) contain calories, and if you eat enough of them, you'll gain weight.

The problem with many carbohydrate foods, including those made from whole grains, is their high glycemic index. The glycemic index was developed by food scientists in the 1980s to compare the effect of different foods on blood sugar levels within two to three hours of consumption.

Before the glycemic index was developed, scientists assumed that table sugar, corn syrup, honey, fructose, and other simple sugars reached the bloodstream much faster than complex carbohydrates such as whole grains, raw fruits, and whole vegetables. Simple sugars were blamed for abrupt changes in blood sugar levels, while complex carbohydrates were considered safer because they were believed to be more gradually absorbed into the bloodstream. Instead, researchers discovered that many foods reach the blood more quickly than plain table sugar does. The foods highest on the glycemic index are dates and parsnips, followed (in this order) by sports drinks, instant rice, puffed rice, jelly beans,

Rice Chex, white rice, pretzels, baked potatoes, instant mashed potatoes, Rice Krispies, cornflakes, rice cakes, Life Savers, jams and jellies, watermelon, wheat crackers, french fries, pumpkin, corn chips, rutabaga, graham crackers, Cheerios, bagels, whole-wheat bread, white bread, saltine crackers, millet, pancakes, and waffles. All of these foods contain sugars that reach the bloodstream faster than plain table sugar, which follows pancakes and waffles on the glycemic index. These foods can cause fatigue, mood swings, and irritability, disrupt body chemistry, and make it difficult or impossible for some individuals to lose weight.

There are so many popular diets, both for weight loss and for improved health, that hundreds of diet books are published every year. Every one of them works for someone, and none of them works for everyone. Your perfect diet is one that fuels your body with the nutrients it needs (which may be very different from the nutrients that someone else requires), leaves you feeling satisfied, and restores your body to perfect health.

Here are some popular as well as little-known diets that have helped many reach that elusive goal.

The Pritikin and Ornish Diets

In the 1960s, Nathan Pritikin was told that his obstructed arteries would kill him within weeks. An engineer and inventor, he decided to look for a cure on his own, and he experimented first with food. Pritikin dramatically reduced his intake of fats and proteins, increased his intake of complex carbohydrates, and avoided sugar, alcohol, coffee, and tobacco. His regimen of diet and exercise worked so well that he was soon free of heart disease. He then published a book and opened a clinic, and thousands of followers used his plan to cure not only their circulatory problems and obesity but other illnesses.

Nutritional requirements vary from one person to another, but many Americans consume far more protein than their bodies can utilize. Arthritis and other chronic conditions are often relieved when a low-protein, low-fat, high-carbohydrate diet corrects nutritional imbalances caused by the long-term overconsumption of protein and fat. However, the improved state of health may not last, and if the new diet doesn't meet the person's nutritional needs, other illnesses and disorders can develop.

In 1980, Ann Louise Gittleman became director of nutrition at the Pritikin Longevity Center in Santa Monica, California. In her book *Beyond Pritikin*, she describes how the Pritikin diet forbids not only saturated fats but the use of nuts, seeds, avocados, olives, unrefined vegetable oils, fatty-acid supplements, and fatty fish, thus excluding the most vital sources of essential fats and fat-soluble vitamins. Although most participants experienced significant health improvements during their stay at the Center, many complained that they felt hungry all the time no matter how much they ate, or they gained weight when they tried to follow the diet at home, or they found it too time-consuming and complicated. Gittleman noticed that those who followed the program for a year or more developed vertical ridges on their fingernails, a symptom of nutritional deficiencies and other problems.

Medical research has linked high-carbohydrate, low-fat diets with some illnesses. In 1992, British researchers published a double-blind, randomized crossover study to test the effects of fats and carbohydrates on emphysema. The study showed small dietary changes in the balance of carbohydrates to fats significantly affected exercise tolerance and breathlessness. The more carbohydrates the patients consumed, the worse their symptoms.

In addition, high-carbohydrate diets have been shown to contribute to serious digestive disorders, mental confusion, epilepsy, and psychiatric disorders, as described on pages 54 to 56.

Like the food pyramid and today's fat-free snack foods, the Pritikin diet's abundant use of fruit and grains contributes to candidiasis in those who are susceptible. Its emphasis on grains causes digestive problems for many, and its lack of essential fatty acids and fat-soluble vitamins contributes to a host of health problems as described on page 72.

Unlike Nathan Pritikin, Dean Ornish, M.D., has credentials that impress physicians, so his findings are taken seriously by a medical establishment that dismissed Pritikin's research out of hand. His 1990 book, *Dr. Dean Ornish's Program for Reversing Heart Disease*, describes the effects of a low-fat vegetarian diet combined with exercise and stress reduction on patients with heart disease. The Pritikin diet includes small amounts of animal protein, so the two plans are not identical, but many who follow the Ornish diet experience the same cravings, mood swings, fatigue, depression, indigestion, nutritional imbalances, and irritability that disrupt the lives of many Pritikin followers.

For some of those who follow it, a low-fat, low-protein, high-carbohydrate diet is at least partially successful. For a few days or weeks, a system that was overburdened with animal protein and fat has an opportunity to rest, cleanse itself, and move into a state of balance. As soon as this balance is achieved, the person feels wonderful. Aches and pains disappear, unwanted pounds fall away, abundant energy returns, and feelings of confidence and optimism make the diet, at least temporarily, easy to follow. But if the diet does not provide the correct ratio of protein, fats, and carbohydrates for that person's unique metabolism, those pleasant results are soon replaced by overwhelming cravings and other symptoms.

The Atkins Diet

At the opposite end of the dietary spectrum is Robert Atkins, M.D., whose diet emphasizes fats and animal-source protein while severely restricting carbohydrates. During the plan's induction phase, which is not recommended for children under age twelve, pregnant women, or anyone with severe kidney disease, dieters avoid all fruits, grains, and starchy vegetables while eating all the meat, poultry, eggs, fish, cream, butter, nuts, seeds, and non-starchy vegetables they like. Dr. Atkins recommends the induction phase for a maximum of two weeks unless a patient has a significant amount of weight to lose, in which case it can be safely continued for weeks or months. In the diet's second phase, carbohydrate consumption is increased in 5-gram increments, which slightly slows the rate of weight loss. Additional carbohydrates are added in the diet's final maintenance phase.

Most nutritionists denounce the Atkins diet as dangerous, but it remains popular because so many respond well to it. On this high-fat, high-protein, high-cholesterol, eat-all-you-want plan, thousands of men and women have been thrilled to see their blood pressure and cholesterol levels fall while they enjoy increased energy, positive thoughts, excellent health, and effortless weight loss. Many diabetics have been able to stop taking insulin by following this diet, and it has helped reverse and cure other chronic conditions as well. The diet includes large quantities of water to keep the system flushed and prevent dehydration. Weight loss during the first two weeks is mostly water weight, and those with chronic edema (fluid retention) often experience immediate relief from that symptom.

But the Atkins approach isn't for everyone. Large amounts of animal protein make some people feel energetic until their systems adjust, at which point they begin to feel tense, anxious, easily distracted, and high-strung. In some patients, excessive amounts of animal protein cause or worsen the symptoms of arthritis or gout. Those whose bodies require large amounts of carbohydrates have trouble converting protein and fat into energy, and if they continue on a high-protein, high-fat diet, they can gain weight, lose strength, have trouble maintaining mental focus, and feel depressed and confused. Because the diet is low in fiber, constipation is a common complaint.

Many followers of the Atkins diet and similar plans find their enthusiasm waning after a week or so; the thought of yet another meal of meat, butter, and eggs becomes unpleasant, and they strongly crave bread, sweets, and other carbohydrates.

To help counteract these cravings and prevent nutritional deficiencies, Dr. Atkins developed an extensive line of supplements and diet foods, including high-protein flour substitutes for baking. However, these products contain many ingredients associated with food sensitivities as well as synthetic vitamins, and they are entirely different from whole foods.

There are several popular variations of the Atkins diet, such as the caveman diet, the carbohydrate addict's diet, and the steak lover's diet, all of which emphasize animal-source protein and eliminate or greatly reduce carbohydrates.

In his popular book *Beyond the Zone: Peak Performance for Radiant Health*, which is another variation of the Atkins diet, Brian Scott Peskin recommends unlimited amounts of meat, poultry, fish, eggs, butter, fats, non-starchy vegetables, small amounts of fruit, and only occasional servings of bread or pasta. In addition, to provide essential nutrients missing from the Atkins diet, he recommends a daily supplement of essential fatty acids (EFAs), chelated or bioavailable minerals, and the herbal tonic Essiac tea, described on page 173. This diet, he claims, results in increased energy, a loss of cravings, increased well-being, better hormone balance, increased calm, improved focus and concentration, and improvement in attention deficit disorders (ADDs) and related problems.

Anti-Candida Diets

Carbohydrates feed *Candida albicans*, an organism native to the human digestive tract. In healthy people, candida cells coexist with hundreds of other bacteria, but in many Americans, they proliferate and cause problems. Candidiasis, which is also known as a chronic or systemic yeast infection, is most common among those who have taken antibiotics. Antibiotics kill both harmful and beneficial bacteria, and when beneficial bacteria no longer hold *Candida albicans* in check, it proliferates. Other drugs that increase susceptibility to candida overgrowth include birth control pills, steroid medications, and drugs that suppress the immune system.

Symptoms of candidiasis include chronic fatigue, especially after eating; drowsiness; insomnia; depression; gastrointestinal problems such as bloating, gas, intestinal cramps, chronic diarrhea, constipation, or heartburn; rectal itching; food allergies; hay fever; severe premenstrual syndrome (PMS); impotence; memory loss, confusion, headaches, and mood swings; recurrent fungal infections such as jock itch, athlete's foot, or ringworm; recurrent vaginal or urinary tract infections; thrush; hypersensitivity to chemicals, perfumes, smoke, and other odors; prostatitis; lightheadedness or feeling intoxicated after drinking minimal wine or beer or eating certain foods; and a worsening of symptoms in damp climates, moldy places such as basements, or after eating or drinking foods containing yeast or sugar. In addition, some researchers blame candidiasis for autoimmune diseases, central nervous system imbalances, earaches, respiratory problems, and other illnesses as well.

Several anti-candida diets published in the 1980s and 1990s resemble the Atkins plan. Most exclude all sugars (including sucrose, dextrose, fructose, fruit juices, corn syrup, honey, maple syrup, brown rice syrup, date sugar or syrup, and molasses), dairy products, fruit, starchy vegetables, wine, beer, spirits, grains, fermented foods, vinegar, mushrooms, and foods containing yeast or molds.

For those with candidiasis, the more abrupt this type of dietary change, the more dramatic and uncomfortable the result. With nothing to eat, candida cells starve, which causes a "die-off" reaction. With billions of dead cells to remove, the body's garbage collectors (the lymph system, liver, and organs of elimination) can be overwhelmed, and the patient typically feels unwell for a few days.

Symptoms of detoxification include fatigue, headache, flulike aches and nausea, diarrhea, malodorous breath and perspiration, a thick coating on the tongue, and fuzzy thinking. In most cases, these symptoms along with the symptoms of candidiasis disappear after three to four days. Providing the nutrients needed for healthy detoxification as described on pages 174 to 175 makes this a more comfortable undertaking. Eating small amounts of carbohydrates reduces the severity of detoxification but prolongs the transition to a low-carbohydrate, anti-candida diet.

A high-protein, low-carbohydrate diet may keep *Candida albicans* in check, but it may not provide the nutrients the body requires. For those whose systems are best fueled by carbohydrates, anti-candida diets work well for short periods but are not the perfect lifelong eating plan their proponents advertise. For additional ways of controlling candida, see pages 61 to 62.

Raw Food Diets

The search for health has brought many to raw-food diet plans. Cooking temperatures above 112 to 120 degrees Fahrenheit (44 to 49 degrees Celsius) destroy key nutrients and enzymes in food, transforming it from "live" to "dead." Raw or live food contains all its enzymes, vitamins, minerals, volatile essential oils, plant hormones, bioflavonoids, pigments such as chlorophyll, natural disinfectants, infection fighters, fiber, and other nutrients.

Experiments on the healing effects of raw food are practically unknown in the United States, but the biological clinics of Europe have repeatedly shown that raw foods can cure disease. For most Americans, raw food means salads and that's as far as our imaginations take us. But raw foodists have developed an entire cuisine of surprisingly versatile recipes and preparation methods. Their books contain inspiring collections of recipes and exciting stories about illness and health.

For those with serious health problems, switching from cooked to raw food, or at least significantly increasing the amount of raw food, often marks the beginning of a full recovery. In the 1950s, Ann Wigmore developed a system of healing based on raw, live foods, including sprouts and wheat grass. Today, as a result of her efforts, most large health food stores offer fresh or frozen wheat grass juice as well as "green" powders and supplements. If she hadn't died in her eighties in a kitchen fire, Wigmore would still be lecturing, giving demonstrations, and writing books. Her philosophy continues to be taught at the institutes she founded in Florida and Puerto Rico.

Raw food diets consist of fruits, vegetables, and occasional servings of sprouted grain and legumes. Unless they include raw dairy products, they can be very low in fat and protein. People who have been eating the standard American diet often do spectacularly well on raw foods for several weeks or months, but after feeling wonderful for a while, many begin to experience fatigue, mood swings, irritability, coldness, strong cravings, and other symptoms. Some who try a raw food regimen never feel well; they dislike it from the beginning and complain of feeling cold, hungry, tired, weak, and in pain from digestive problems.

Even if you decide not to experiment with an all-raw diet, some raw foods belong at every meal. In fact, beginning each meal with a taste of raw food as described on page 2 eliminates a stressful reaction caused by cooked foods.

Thanks to raw foodists, those who are otherwise unable to digest grain can enjoy occasional bread without discomfort. Interest in raw-food diets has created a market for Essene, Ezekiel, Manna, or "Bible" bread, which is made entirely of sprouted grain. Sold in health food store freezers, it is a sweet, sticky, dense bread that, unlike regular bread, does not inhibit calcium absorption or cause digestive problems. Sprouting increases the level of B and C vitamins, destroys the enzyme inhibitors found in grains, and destroys a gluten lectin found in the seed coat. Lectins are proteins that can act as antigens and cause allergic reactions (see page 51). A lectin in unsprouted wheat can attach to insulin receptors and interfere with insulin efficiency, while a lectin in unsprouted rye can settle in the vascular system and contribute to blood disorders and circulatory problems.

Juice Fasting

While it's true that Americans don't eat enough fiber, an impaired digestive tract may not be able to cope with a sudden supply of raw produce. Juicing is a popular therapy because juices are concentrated, nutritious, and easy to assimilate. They are, in a sense, predigested. Someone whose stomach and intestines would be overwhelmed by even a few raw vegetables can absorb their nutrients by swallowing fresh vegetable juice. Fresh juices contain all the enzymes and nutrients found in the fruits or vegetables from which they are made. Bottled juices are not recommended because even if they don't contain added sugar, artificial color, or chemical preservatives, they are pasteurized and therefore do not contain the beneficial enzymes and other heat-sensitive nutrients of raw juice.

Juice fasting is a popular therapy in health spas and among people who want to lose weight in a hurry. Consuming nothing but freshly prepared raw juices is an easy way to flush toxins from the system while giving the digestive tract a well-deserved rest. Some raw-juice therapies include wheat grass juice, herbal teas, and various herbal or nutritional supplements. Such programs have been credited with curing serious illnesses, including cancer, heart disease, and rheumatoid and osteoarthritis.

Juice fasting is safe for most people for short periods, such as a few days at a time. Therapeutic juice fasts, which are used to treat specific illnesses, should be supervised by an experienced health care professional. Fruit juices and sweet vegetable juices, such as carrot juice, are high on the glycemic index and can cause abrupt changes in blood sugar levels as well as worsen candida yeast infections.

Some nutritionists argue that juicing is unhealthy because it's unnatural. No one eats 5 pounds of apples in one sitting, but it's easy to drink the juice of that many apples in a few minutes. Consuming so many concentrated nutrients may be dangerous, the critics claim. Juice therapists counter by saying that people with impaired digestion, which includes most Americans, cannot digest all the nutrients in even a single apple. By releasing the nutrients in raw foods, juicing makes them easy to assimilate. For those with serious digestive problems, juices may be too concentrated for comfort. In those cases, any change of diet is best approached gradually. Start with small amounts, say the experts; dilute juice with water and increase quantities as your system adjusts.

Another objection is that juicing removes fiber from the diet. Someone eating a raw carrot consumes not only its digestible parts but its indigestible roughage. Juice therapists explain that just as too much juice too soon can be detrimental, too much fiber can overwhelm the system and cause a different set of problems. Raw salads containing small amounts of grated carrot, other fibrous vegetables, raw apples including the skin, and similar sources of fiber provide the bulk that is necessary for good intestinal health while allowing the system to adjust without complications.

Juice fasting and raw food diets work best when they feature the fruits and vegetables that are most compatible with a person's body chemistry, as described in chapter 3.

Food Combining

Advocates of food combining believe that all diets create problems when people eat without regard to the way foods interact with each other and with the digestive tract. According to this theory, fruits should be eaten alone for breakfast or between meals because the body digests them faster than other foods, while protein (only one type is allowed per meal) should be eaten with leafy green vegetables, and other vegetables should be eaten alone or with grains or legumes. Fruits and vegetables should never be combined; neither should dairy products and meat, or starches and citrus fruit. Harvey and Marilyn Diamond's book *Fit for Life* introduced the concepts of food combining to an international audience.

The basic rules of food combining, which can be adapted to any diet, have helped many people improve their digestion. Can you ignore these guidelines and still enjoy perfect digestion? Yes, especially if your diet is perfectly matched to your body chemistry and your digestive system is basically healthy. Also, food combining will not change your body's chemistry, so that if you require large amounts of protein, a correctly combined grain-based diet won't feed you correctly. For those who don't utilize carbohydrates well, eating fruit by itself disrupts blood sugar levels and leads to fatigue, confusion, physical weakness, and other unpleasant symptoms.

It is important to find one's own optimum mix of proteins, fats, and carbohydrates before dwelling on the combinations.

Macrobiotics

The macrobiotic diet introduced to America by George Ohsawa in the late 1950s is based on a traditional Japanese diet. Whole grains and vegetables make up 75 to 90 percent of this almost-vegetarian, no-fruit diet, with the rest consisting of sea vegetables, nuts, seeds, fermented soy products, salty condiments, occasional fish or eggs, and roasted Japanese twig tea. To accommodate cravings for sweets, which are common on this regimen, barley malt, rice syrup, and maple syrup or candies made from them are allowed on special occasions.

As successful as it is for many of its followers, the macrobiotic approach is often applied as strictly as the Pritikin and Ornish "prescription" diets, with similar results. In her excellent book *Food and Healing*, Annemarie Colbin describes how the macrobiotic diet, which has cured many cases of cancer and other serious illnesses, can be adjusted to prevent out-of-control cravings, fatigue, and mood swings by increasing the amount of fish, beans, and salad; adding fruit to the menu; using grains other than brown rice; decreasing the overall proportion of grains and salty condiments; and by seasoning foods with otherwise forbidden herbs and spices.

Once a strict follower of macrobiotic rules, Colbin has adopted a more flexible "health-supportive whole-foods eating style." Her book and its companion cookbook, *The Natural Gourmet*, offer nutritional insights that are grounded in common sense and based on the experiences of hundreds of students, friends, and family members. Her recommendation is a daily diet comprised of 20 to 25 percent fats, 10 to 12 percent protein, and 70 to 75 percent carbohydrates, but these proportions are only suggestions.

In the 1970s, Colbin thrived on a vegan diet, which is free of all animal products. However, her husband, a gourmet macrobiotic chef, grew thin, cold, depressed, fatigued, and unhealthy-looking on the same foods. Believing he was going through a healing crisis, he persevered for another ten months before adding more whole grains, beans, and fish to his diet. This helped, but he still felt unwell, with low moods and matching energy levels.

When her husband described his strong craving for steak, Colbin encouraged him to try some. Even though it disagreed with their vegetarian philosophy, he took her advice and felt immediately better. Gradually, he began eating fish or poultry almost daily and steak once a week, and his health and energy returned. As Colbin writes, "John's experience was a lesson for both of us about the fallacy of being stuck in any single, strict food ideology." She recites similar examples of people who pursued a strict regimen for philosophical reasons even though it impaired their health.

WE ARE NOT ALL ALIKE

There is no single perfect diet that works for everyone, and a one-size-fits-all mentality is the major shortcoming of the government-endorsed food pyramid, the Pritikin, Ornish, and Atkins diets, raw food diets, the macrobiotic diet, and every other diet that assumes that all humans have the same nutritional requirements.

Cravings are symptoms of inadequate nutrition. The most extreme cravings, resulting from a condition called *pica*, accompany severe mineral deficiencies; people with pica are known to eat charcoal, laundry starch, pebbles, and other non-food items. Less dramatic but just as indicative of nutritional imbalances is binge eating.

Someone whose intake of nutrients exactly matches the needs of her body will feel hungry when it's time to eat, but that person won't be overwhelmed by cravings.

A diet may be perfectly balanced on paper, but if the body can't digest and absorb its nutrients, deficiencies will result. For example, phytic acid in grains and legumes binds with calcium, iron, magnesium, phosphorus, and zinc in the intestinal tract, preventing their absorption. Wheat, oats, and soy have the highest concentrations of phytates. In large amounts, phytates can cause mineral deficiencies, bone loss, intestinal distress, and allergies. Cooking does not destroy phytates, but soaking does. It is interesting that traditional cultures around the world soaked their grains and legumes for several hours or overnight before cooking them. Fermentation destroys phytates, too. Because they are fermented, miso, tempeh, natto, and shoyu (soy sauce) do not contain phytates, but soy milk, tofu, soy protein, soy nuts, soy yogurt, and all other soy foods do. It's easy to see how someone whose system doesn't digest carbohydrates well can suffer from more than simple indigestion on a diet based on grains and soy foods.

Weston Price's research showed that people around the world developed healthful but entirely different diets depending on climate and the availability of food. It is a serious mistake to insist, as most physicians and dietitians do, that the same basic diet is ideal for all. The old adage that one man's meat is another man's poison is literally true.

Growing up in an isolated culture that has emphasized the same foods for hundreds or thousands of years makes menu selection easy, and those who use their ancestors' traditional ingredients and preparation techniques even when they live modern lives can maintain excellent health in the twenty-first century. Even people who don't tolerate carbohydrates well often benefit from whatever grain their ancestors ate, such as rice among Asians and rye among Scandinavians. In the United States today, uninterrupted pedigrees are rare.

Most of us are so genetically diverse it's difficult to know which if any culture's traditional fare will work for us. Our body chemistries may be the best predictors of our ideal diets.

The Blood-Type Diet

The first best-selling book to present menu plans based on individual body chemistries was *Eat Right 4 Your Type* by Peter J. D'Adamo, N.D. A naturopathic physician, Dr. D'Adamo realized that the four human blood types offer far more information than which type to use when giving a transfusion. "Each of the four blood types," he explains, "evolved in response to both the physiologic development of the species and changing climatic conditions over the eons." These evolutionary changes affected how the immune system coped with unfamiliar bacteria, viruses, and environmental factors, and at the same time allowed the digestive system to adapt to unfamiliar foods.

According to Dr. D'Adamo, type O, the oldest and most common blood type worldwide, dates back to Cro-Magnons, whose primary food was meat. The original hunter-gatherer, type O does best on an animal protein-based diet. Type A, which developed 17,000 to 27,000 years ago, accompanied an increased consumption of plants, grains, and fish as people settled in permanent communities. Type B, which developed 12,000 to 17,000 years ago, evolved as a more balanced blood chemistry than either of its predecessors as people left settled areas and became nomads. This type thrived on the meat and milk of cattle, sheep, and goats as well as everything that could be scavenged, and developed a truly omnivorous diet. An estimated ten to fifteen centuries ago, the very rare type AB emerged. Its purpose is not yet known, says D'Adamo, but it incorporates the strengths and weaknesses of both types A and B.

In 1996, when D'Adamo's book was published, most physicians and nutritionists dismissed it as unproven and unscientific. However, some published research on blood chemistry and its effect on digestion supports his theory. Many nutritionally oriented physicians are testing it on their patients with good to excellent results. According to Peter D'Adamo:

- Type O's ideal diet is high in protein, and includes meat, poultry, fish, and a variety of fruits and vegetables. Grains, legumes (including soy), dairy products, alcohol, and sugar are incompatible with type O.
- Type A's ideal diet is primarily vegetarian, and includes soy products, beans, legumes, grains, vegetables, and fruits, with small portions of fish. Dairy products are incompatible with type A.
- Type B's ideal diet includes game meats such as venison and rabbit as well as herd meats, such as lamb and mutton. Unlike types O and A, type B benefits from different kinds of dairy products. Although some grains, beans, and legumes cause problems for this type, it has by far the most varied diet.
- Type AB's ideal diet is primarily vegetarian with small, occasional servings of meat and fermented milk products such as yogurt and kefir. This type, D'Adamo says, should avoid chicken.

It is easy to discover your blood type using a home testing kit (see Resources) or by visiting a blood donation center. The blood-type theory deserves credit for calling attention to human chemical differences, which helps explain why no single diet works well for everyone.

Does it work? Some type Os thrive on a vegetarian diet despite D'Adamo's claim that they can't derive protein from plants. Not all type Os do well on animal protein, and some type As live long, healthy lives on dairy products even though their blood type is supposed to be incompatible with cow's milk.

If the blood-type theory is fundamentally sound, acculturation may explain these deviations from the norm. Individuals have adjusted to life in very different cultures for millennia, and after several generations, their descendants were well adapted to a diet very different from the one their blood type evolved on.

The Metabolic Typing Diet

Four years after *Eat Right 4 Your Type* was published, William L. Wolcott took individual diets a step further by publishing *The Metabolic Typing Diet*. Metabolic typing defines one's body chemistry, compares it to specific foods, and creates a perfectly matched diet.

The history of metabolic typing is a fascinating tale of medical puzzle solving, which Wolcott recounts in detail. This system of medicine disregards conventional diagnoses because the underlying cause of every illness is a lack of whatever nutrients the patient's body requires. What matters is not a person's medical history, lab test results, prescription drugs, or symptoms, but rather his unique metabolic type and its nutritional requirements. Two patients may present exactly the same symptoms, but the diets that cure them can be polar opposites. For example, one man with hypertension was defined as having parasympathetic dominance, fast oxidation, and anabolic imbalance. He improved quickly on a high-protein, high-fat diet with no supplements. Another man with identical symptoms showed sympathetic dominance, catabolic imbalance, and electrolyte excess. He was cured by a low-fat, low-protein, high-carbohydrate diet with some supplemental nutrients.

Much has been written in macrobiotic and other diet books about the importance of acid/alkaline balance, but as Wolcott points out, even pH reactions to food are individual. In the autonomic-dominant type, vegetables have an alkalinizing effect while meats acidify the system, but in the oxidative-dominant type, the opposite is true. Contrary to conventional wisdom, he explains, no food or nutrient has an inherently acid or alkaline effect on the body. Instead, its interaction with the various fundamental homeostatic controls of different metabolic types determines whether a food will have an alkaline or acid effect.

Peter D'Adamo agrees, stating that type A performs best when the body tissues are slightly alkaline, in contrast to type O, which performs best when slightly acid. The same food can have an alkaline reaction in one system and an acid reaction in another, such as the inner kernel of wheat, which is alkaline in type O and acidic in type A.

Wolcott's book includes a simplified version of the questionnaire his clinic uses to determine metabolic types. It measures irritability, anxiety, or fatigue in response to different foods; weather preferences; coughing spells; cravings; dandruff; ear color; eating habits; favorite foods; gag reflex; nose moisture; saliva quantity; stamina; eye pupil size; and other factors. The questionnaire reveals three basic metabolic diets: protein, carbohydrate, and mixed protein/carbohydrate. Each metabolic type has subdivisions that further individualize menu planning.

Wolcott uses blood types not as indicators of what to eat but of what foods to avoid. Proteins called lectins are found in small quantities in about one-third of all foods. Although cooking and the digestive process inhibit their activity to some extent, many enter the bloodstream, where they act as antigens, or foreign invaders. Different lectins bind to the surfaces of different blood cells.

According to Wolcott, lectins often cause clumping and the subsequent destruction of blood cells, and their interference with digestion and absorption causes additional problems such as nutritional deficiencies, food allergies, inflammatory bowel disease, diabetes mellitus, rheumatoid arthritis, psoriasis, infertility, flatulence, immune deficiencies, fatigue, headache, body aches, diarrhea, irritability, and anemia.

"The good news," he says, "is that many lectins are blood-type specific, which means that they can cause negative effects in people with specific blood types."

According to Wolcott:

- Blood type A should avoid blackberries, brown trout, clams, cornflakes, French mushrooms (*Hygrophorus hypothejus*), halibut, flounder, lima beans, snow-white mushrooms, sole, soybeans, soybean sprouts, string beans, tora beans, and the breakfast cereals Total and Product 19.
- Blood type B should avoid bitter pear melons, black-eyed peas, chicken, chocolate, cocoa, French mushrooms (*Hygrophorus hypothejus* and *Marasmius orcades*), pomegranates, salmon, sesame seeds, sunflower seeds, soybeans, and tuna.

- Blood type AB should avoid blackberries, black-eyed peas, brown trout, clams, cocoa, cornflakes, French mushrooms (*Hygrophorus hypothejus*), halibut, flounder, lima beans, pomegranates, salmon, sesame seeds, snow-white mushrooms, sole, soybeans, soybean sprouts, string beans, sunflower seeds, tuna, Product 19, and Total.
- Blood type O should avoid blackberries, chocolate, cocoa, French mushrooms (*Amanita muscaria*), halibut, flounder, sole, and sunflower seeds.

The importance of eating to satisfy the needs of your individual body cannot be over emphasized. In *The Metabolic Typing Diet*, Wolcott describes the adventures of Carl Zander, starting middle linebacker for the Cincinnati Bengals in the 1989 Super Bowl. Zander phoned Wolcott from training camp in 1990 because he was mysteriously losing muscle mass all over his body and, with it, the ability to burn fat. He had been in peak condition just a few weeks before, and now he was losing strength, endurance, speed, reaction time, and agility. His recovery from bruises and contusions had slowed, and he suffered from extreme fatigue during and after practice. He knew he would soon lose his starting position and asked for any help Wolcott could offer.

A complete metabolic evaluation usually takes two weeks, but Zander couldn't wait that long, so they discussed his dietary history. He sounded like a parasympathetic dominant, which is the type that needs the most protein, and the breakthrough came when Zander mentioned that his training camp coaches were enthusiastic advocates of carbohydrate loading. Before practice every day, players were encouraged to eat substantial quantities of carbohydrates to sustain their energy. Wolcott suggested that Zander ignore that advice and, while his teammates ate pasta and bagels, eat all the red meat and butter he could. Because so many experts warned against the dangers of red meat, cholesterol, and saturated fat, this was unexpected advice, but Zander was desperate enough to try it.

His fatigue disappeared almost immediately, his muscle tissue began to restore itself, and his metabolic rate increased along with his ability to recover rapidly from bruises, muscle strains, and other injuries.

Meanwhile, many of Zander's teammates thrived on the same diet that had caused him to gain weight and deteriorate. "I see this metabolic diversity among athletes all the time," says Wolcott. A few years before meeting Zander, Wolcott worked with a former National Football League quarterback who had gained weight on a high-protein diet. He experienced all the symptoms that would later plague Zander, but in reverse. Because he wasn't getting adequate glucose from carbohydrates, this man's body was catabolizing or tearing down his muscle tissue for the fuel it desperately needed. Adrenal and thyroid imbalances further contributed to his fatigue and sluggishness, and as his metabolic rate slowed, he began to store fat rather than burn it.

The retired quarterback adopted a low-protein, high-carbohydrate diet on which he quickly regained energy and muscle strength. In addition, although he ate whatever he wanted and never deprived himself of his favorite foods, he lost nearly 2 pounds per week for eight months.

Clinical trials designed to settle the argument about which diet works best, such as a comparison between the Ornish and Atkins diets, can never reach anything but inconclusive results. Unless participants are selected according to their body chemistries, some dieters will succeed and others will fail no matter how carefully they follow the diet's guidelines.

It will be years before the concept of dieting according to body chemistry is adopted by mainstream medicine. In the meantime, you can become acquainted with your own unique requirements and in the process become a nutritional expert.

The Specific Carbohydrate Diet

Carbohydrates cause serious health problems for many, but an inability to digest carbohydrates may be temporary rather than lifelong. After following a therapeutic diet to repair the digestive tract, many carbohydrate-intolerant patients are able to consume carbohydrates with good results.

The most extreme example of carbohydrate intolerance is celiac sprue or celiac disease, a chronic disorder of the small intestine caused by an inability to digest carbohydrates and gluten. Celiac disease interferes with the body's absorption of fat, protein, carbohydrates, iron, water, and vitamins A, D, E, and K. Found mostly in people of northwestern European ancestry, celiac disease is several times more common in Ireland than in the United States. Symptoms usually begin in childhood with the introduction of wheat cereal or other foods containing gluten, but they can be triggered by other carbohydrates as well. Symptoms include painful bloating, stunted growth, iron deficiency anemia, bone deformation, and pale, bulky, malodorous stools. In some cases, symptoms disappear during adolescence and reappear in adulthood.

Most physicians prescribe a gluten-free, high-protein, low-fat diet for celiac disease. When that approach fails, patients typically blame themselves for not being sufficiently vigilant, blame the manufacturers of gluten-free products for accidental gluten contamination, or simply feel depressed, discouraged, and exhausted.

A far more effective remedy is the specific carbohydrate diet described by Elaine Gottschall in her book *Breaking the Vicious Cycle: Intestinal Health Through Diet.* Gottschall learned about the specific carbohydrate diet in 1958, when she took her eight-year-old daughter to Drs. Sidney V. and Merrill P. Haas, who were famous for curing hundreds of cases of celiac disease and cystic fibrosis of the pancreas using diet alone. After following the specific carbohydrate diet for a year or more, patients were able to return to a normal diet with a complete and permanent disappearance of symptoms.

Gottschall's daughter had already received three years of conventional treatment with cortisone, sulfonamides, and other medical therapies, but her condition had deteriorated so much that surgery seemed imminent. On the specific carbohydrate diet, she recovered and within two years was free of symptoms. After another few years, she returned to a normal diet and has since remained in excellent health.

The specific carbohydrate diet cures not only all types of celiac disease but ulcerative colitis, Crohn's disease, diverticulitis, and other causes of chronic diarrhea, as well as schizophrenia, cystic fibrosis of the pancreas, epilepsy, mental confusion, poor memory, bizarre behavior, autistic-type hypoactivity, hyperactivity, severe and prolonged night terrors, and wasting diseases caused by the malabsorption of nutrients. When Gottschall's daughter was cured of ulcerative colitis, the first symptoms to disappear were delirious seizures that occurred in her sleep several times weekly. Throughout the twentieth century, researchers studying the brain-bowel connection concluded that many psychoses and neuroses are reactions to biological factors that are digestive in nature, and that schizophrenia is the result of chronic intoxication from psychotoxic factors produced in the intestine.

The vicious cycle described by Gottschall's title refers to impaired digestion of disaccharides (the carbohydrates maltose, lactose, sucrose, and others), which results in their malabsorption, which triggers bacterial overgrowth, which increases bacterial by-products and mucus production, which injures the surface of the small intestine, which further impairs the digestion of disaccharides.

The specific carbohydrate diet excludes all starches, sugars, and grains, most beans, and all dairy products except a specific type of dry curd cottage cheese and homemade yogurt that ferments for twenty-four hours before being used. Protein foods, non-starchy vegetables, nuts, fats, and specific fruits are its main foods. Honey, a monosaccharide, is allowed in small amounts. This diet, which requires careful planning and diligent label reading, frees patients of debilitating symptoms and restores them to good health and confident, active lives.

CHAPTER THREE

Creating the Custom Diet

As CHAPTER 2 EXPLAINS, IT IS impossible to find a diet that works for everyone, and any effort to comply with specific ratios of carbohydrates, protein, fats, vitamins, minerals, and other nutrients is an exercise in futility unless it's based on body chemistry.

As you experiment with your diet, stay away from canned, fried, microwaved, irradiated, and processed food as much as possible. Replace white flour, sugar, bottled juices, and other convenience foods with whole grains, fresh fruits, and vegetables. Buy the best meat, poultry, eggs, and dairy products you can, preferably organically raised from free-range animals.

Here are some ways to fine-tune your diet.

FOOD SENSITIVITIES
AND HOW TO TEST FOR THEM

There is much debate and confusion over the term *food allergy.* To orthodox physicians, an allergic reaction is immediate and dramatic, like anaphylactic shock, which can be fatal, or a sudden eruption of hives. The term *food sensitivity* was coined to describe more subtle reactions that also may be debilitating.

Although there are blood tests and patch tests designed to detect food allergies and sensitivities, you can conduct your own effective test at home with pencil in hand. Keep a notebook of everything you eat, when you eat it, how your body responds, and how you feel. Sometimes this simple exercise will bring to light an obvious connection between cause and symptom.

A more serious test is the four-day rotation diet. Because it takes four days for the body to remove all traces of the food consumed, this system schedules four days of menus according to related food groups. On day one you might eat wheat, then no wheat at all on days two, three, and four. If you eat eggs today, don't eat them again for four days, and don't eat chicken, either, because it comes from the same animal.

The four-day rotation diet is time consuming and requires careful planning. You have to read labels constantly, and it's impossible to dine out unless you avoid sauces and salad dressings, check ingredients with your waiter or hostess, and write everything down as you consume it. Unless you can verify their food sources and other ingredients, stop taking vitamins and food supplements. Beverages can cause all kinds of complications. Forget Coke and Pepsi. Nearly all "healthy" soft drinks, bottled iced tea, and bottled juice blends contain high-fructose corn syrup. If they contain sugar, is it from beets or sugar cane? Beer contains barley, malt, hops, and yeast, and that's if you buy a German beer or a brand that lists its ingredients. American beers are notorious for sudsing agents, artificial colors, preservatives, and chemical additives that never appear on labels.

After you've followed this regimen for a week, start rearranging foods so that you test different combinations. Keep food families in mind. On the day you drink soy milk, you can eat tofu, tempeh, soy sauce, miso, and any other soy product. For the next three days, avoid all soy foods. On the day you eat tomatoes, eat all you want of eggplant, peppers, and potatoes, as all are members of the nightshade family—then avoid eating any of these "cousin" foods for three days. Tobacco, by the way, also is a nightshade.

For a detailed description of rotation testing and a complete list of food families, check for books in your library or health food store, such as *If This Is Tuesday, It Must Be Chicken: Or How to Rotate Your Food for Better Nutrition* by N. Golos and F. Golbitz.

Another way to test for food sensitivities is by taking your pulse. This simple procedure was discovered fifty years ago by Arthur M. Coca, M.D., founder of the *Journal of Immunology* and a highly regarded research scientist. Coca's breakthrough was simplicity itself. If you eat a food that agrees with you, your pulse rate will remain stable. If you eat one that doesn't, your pulse will increase. In his medical practice and through his book *The Pulse Test,* Coca trained thousands to monitor their diets and make their own accurate diagnoses.

In order to take the pulse test accurately, you must stop smoking for the duration of the test and be free of conditions that might disrupt your pulse, such as fighting off a cold or being sunburned.

Count your pulse for sixty seconds just after waking in the morning and just before going to bed at night. In addition, take it just before each meal and again thirty minutes, sixty minutes, and ninety minutes after the meal ends. Always take your pulse sitting up, except when you first wake up in the morning, and count your heartbeats for a full minute.

Keep a food journal for two or three days, noting everything you eat at each meal and the day's pulse rates. Some connections may be obvious at once. If your pulse jumps from 65 beats per minute just before breakfast to 85 beats per minute after, something in the French toast may not agree with you. One woman discovered that her pulse raced every morning just after she got up. After three days of record keeping, she realized that the problem was her toothpaste. When she changed brands, her chronic migraine headaches disappeared.

You can use the pulse test to check individual foods and narrow your findings to a single offender. Eliminate foods that cause your pulse to race and you'll eliminate health problems with them.

What if giving up your favorite food makes you feel worse? That's not uncommon. Just as people who give up tobacco, coffee, or alcohol go through withdrawal symptoms, so do many who give up wheat, dairy products, or other foods. Because our bodies are accustomed to the foods we eat every day or several times a day, the absence of those foods may generate headaches, fatigue, diarrhea, or other symptoms of detoxification. These symptoms are most likely to occur when a dramatic change is made suddenly. For more on detoxification, see pages 171 to 176.

INTESTINAL BACTERIA

If you live in America, the odds are you have taken antibiotics. These powerful and overused drugs take a toll on a healthy body. In addition to other side effects, they destroy our intestines' beneficial bacteria. Healthy intestinal microflora typically contain between four hundred and five hundred different species of bacteria, most of them in the colon. Important supporters of the immune system, these bacteria produce enzymes, improve digestion, lower the risk of irritable bowel syndrome, inhibit the growth of pathogens, prevent diarrhea, synthesize vitamins, detoxify the body, and protect against toxins.

Because antibiotics destroy beneficial as well as harmful bacteria, antibiotic treatment is often followed by gastrointestinal discomfort, diarrhea, incomplete digestion, a susceptibility to yeast or fungal infections, (such as *Candida albicans*) and lowered immunity. According to some researchers, imbalances of intestinal bacteria can cause chronic fatigue, fibromyalgia, irritable bowel syndrome, flatulence, constipation, susceptibility to colds and flu, poor immune response, chronic bladder infections, allergies, skin problems, the rapid onset of osteoporosis, high cholesterol levels, vitamin B deficiencies, food sensitivities, menstrual complaints, and chronic bad breath.

Fortunately, beneficial bacteria can be replaced. Several types are grown in laboratories for use in supplements, including *Lactobacillus acidophilus, L. bulgaricus, L. rhamnosus, L. casei, L. plantarum, Streptococcus faecium, S. thermophilus, Bifidobacterium bifidum,* and other strains with imposing names. These bacteria have an ancient history, for people have been using them to culture soured milk foods for centuries. Lactic acid is the common by-product of the fermentation of milk from cows, goats, sheep, camels, and mares; it breaks down fat, sugar, and proteins to make the milk more digestible.

Cultured milk dishes are always best when freshly made, when their taste is superior and their bacteria most lively. Unfortunately, even friendly bacteria can be enemies. As yogurt ages, its *L. acidophilus* competes with *L. bulgaricus* and the result can be dead acidophilus long before the carton's expiration date.

To invite beneficial bacteria back into your system:

- Make your own yogurt using a commercial yogurt starter (see Resources), acidophilus powder, or a probiotic powder containing different strains of beneficial bacteria.
- Buy acidophilus powder or supplements from your health food store's refrigerated section (look for blue or

amber glass jars with distant expiration dates) or by mail, and sprinkle it on food. Take before breakfast, when stomach acid is less concentrated, or just after a meal, when food acts as a buffer. Some acidophilus capsules and tablets are designed to break down later in the digestive process, and a few brands claim to survive stomach acid.

Bifudus strains are native to humans and will reproduce in the intestines over time. Some brands contain a single strain of bacteria, while others, such as Flora Source probiotic powder, contain as many as fourteen different strains. Opinions differ as to which approach is better, but considering the hundreds of different strains that coexist in healthy humans, it makes sense to restore as many types of beneficial bacteria as possible.

- Feed your friendly bacteria. In his book *Acidophilus and Colon Health: The Natural Way to Prevent Disease,* David Webster reports that most Americans, even those who have taken prescription antibiotics several times, have at least some surviving acidophilus and bifidus bacteria. All these bacteria need, he says, is the right kind of food and a system that is slightly acidic rather than alkaline. Webster recommends sweet whey as the ideal food for intestinal bacteria; other experts use fructooligosaccharides (FOS) supplements, lactic-acid fermented vegetables such as unpasteurized sauerkraut, or the Swiss liquid-whey concentrate Molkosan, which is appropriate for those who are lactose-intolerant because it does not contain milk solids. As Webster points out, supplements consisting of isolated whey protein do not feed beneficial bacteria.

Onions and cabbage are reported to be good for these friendly microbes, as is dextrose, a sugar found in rice and corn. The tubers of Jerusalem artichokes, also called sunchokes because they are members of the sunflower family, contain inulin, a favorite food of lactobacteria. Popular in Japan as a food for intestinal health, Jerusalem artichoke flour is available in U.S. health food stores, and the raw tubers are sold in many supermarkets.

LACTO-FERMENTED VEGETABLES

A simple way to improve the digestibility of vegetables while supporting beneficial bacteria is with lactic acid fermentation. Lactic acid is what turns milk into yogurt and transforms cabbage into sauerkraut. It is a natural preservative, but it does much more than make food last longer. Lactic acid produces vitamin C, vitamin B_{12}, enzymes that support metabolic activity, choline, which balances and nourishes the blood, and acetylcholine, which tones the nerves, calms the mind, and improves sleep patterns. Lactic acid is also a chemical repressor that fights cancer cells without harming healthy cells. In Europe and Asia, lacto-fermented vegetables have long been staple foods. Now they are a cancer therapy as well.

As William L. Fischer explains in his book *How to Fight Cancer and Win*, unpasteurized sauerkraut and other fermented vegetables are living foods that improve bowel health and digestion, maintain beneficial intestinal flora, help eliminate harmful bacteria, improve the assimilation of nutrients, prevent chronic conditions from developing, and enhance healing.

To make lacto-fermented vegetables, you don't need special equipment, although a Japanese salad press or German pickle crock simplifies the effort (see Resources). You can make them in a glass or ceramic bowl using a plate to press the vegetables. The basic ingredients are vegetables, a pinch of salt, a few optional herbs, and time. Cucumbers, the fastest to prepare, are ready in about two hours. Carrots and other root vegetables take a couple of days if they are sliced rather than shredded, and a week or more if prepared in a large ceramic crock.

Vegetables are ready when they taste tangy and feel slightly soft. They keep well, for weeks or months, refrigerated in tightly sealed glass jars.

For best results, use an unrefined sea salt such as Eden, Lima, or Celtic Sea Salt, all of which are sold in health food stores (see Resources). Salt helps break down the vegetables' outer cell wall, draws out excess water, and concentrates the vegetables' nutrients. Alternatively, use a salty condiment, such as shoyu, miso, or umeboshi plum paste.

Wash vegetables thoroughly to remove sand, but do not peel organically grown produce except for thick-skinned cucumbers; if the vegetables are commercially grown, reduce pesticide residues by washing well, removing outer leaves, or peeling. Then slice with a knife, grate or shred with a grater, or puree, slice or shred with a food processor, discarding any tough stems or damaged portions.

Use only glass, ceramic, stainless steel, or plastic pressing materials, not aluminum, tin, or copper. Keep all utensils meticulously clean.

The following recipes are suggestions only. Use any vegetables that are handy. Raw beans contain enzymes that interfere with fermentation and should be simmered for five minutes in boiling water before pressing; all other vegetables should be raw. Vegetables that are dry rather than juicy can be helped with a "starter" of liquid from a previous batch. If such a starter is unavailable, you can add a small amount of Molkosan liquid whey (a concentrated source of lactic acid) mixed with an equal quantity of plain water.

Too busy to make your own? Some health food stores carry lacto-fermented vegetables, including unpasteurized sauerkraut (see Resources).

Cucumbers in an Open Bowl

Slice peeled cucumbers up to ¼ inch thick. Find a plate that will just fit inside the bowl; it will be your press. Fill a large jar with water; it will be your weight. To each firmly packed cup of cucumber slices, add ⅛ teaspoon sea salt. Fill the bowl almost to the top with the cucumber slices, cover with the plate, and weight it with the jar.

If using a Japanese salad press, combine 8 cups of cucumber slices with 1 teaspoon salt, fill the press, attach the lid, and screw the pressing plate down firmly. In about two hours (more or less, depending on the thickness of the slices and the temperature of the room), juice will cover the plate and your cucumbers will be tangy, crisp, and ready to eat.

Pressed Salad

Shred or finely mince any combination of greens or cabbage (Chinese, green, or purple cabbage, beet greens, turnip greens, dandelion greens, etc.); grate, thinly slice, or julienne carrots, radishes, parsnips, beets, green peppers, parsley, scallions, and/or other colorful vegetables. Mix 8 cups of firmly packed vegetables with 1 teaspoon sea salt, 2 cloves minced garlic, and 1 to 2 teaspoons minced fresh herbs or ½ to 1 teaspoon dried herbs (sage, rosemary, thyme, dill, basil, oregano, etc.).

If using an open bowl, crush, knead, or mix until the vegetables begin to soften; fill the bowl as described above, and press until ready. If using a plastic salad press, simply stir to mix well, fill the press, fasten the lid, screw the top down tightly (but not so tightly that you break the mechanism), and after two to three hours, tighten it a bit more. The vegetables will compress as they ferment.

If brine does not cover the vegetables within two hours at normal room temperature (65 to 75 degrees Fahrenheit), your vegetables need more crushing, more salt, or a heavier weight. Press for up to six hours or overnight. In hot weather, the vegetables may be ready much sooner; in cold weather, press for up to twenty-four hours.

To make a larger version of this salad, shred or cut enough vegetables to pack a ceramic German pickle crock three-quarters full, and mix with an appropriate amount of sea salt (1 tablespoon salt per 24 cups of vegetables). The crock comes with heavy stone weights to keep the vegetables submerged, and the top has a special lip that seals the lid when its deep groove is filled with water. This one-way water seal allows gases to escape from within while protecting the vegetables from exposure to air and preventing the development of a frothy scum that would otherwise require removal. Depending on how finely you cut or shred the vegetables, the process may take one week or, for coarsely cut vegetables, up to four weeks or longer.

For more detailed instructions, see *Making Sauerkraut and Pickled Vegetables at Home: The Original Lactic Acid Fermentation Method* by Annelies Schoeneck. Try to consume at least some lacto-fermented vegetables every day. They can be used as salad ingredients, garnishes, or condiments. You can cook with them, too, but remember that heating foods above body temperature destroys nutrients, so experiment with recipes and try adding lacto-fermented vegetables just before serving.

DIGESTING GRAINS

In the industrial West, grain is taken from field to storage in a single day. This is very different from traditional harvesting methods, in which cut grain was left in the field for days or weeks, during which rain and sunlight provided the conditions needed for germination. In traditional cultures around the world, grain was ground just before use and soaked overnight before cooking. Gruels and porridges were cooked slowly over gentle heat, and breads were allowed to ferment for days before baking. All of these steps increased the vitamins, enzymes, amino acids, and other nutrients in grain while removing chemicals that interfere with digestion.

According to Sally Fallon, founder of the Weston A. Price Foundation and author of the seminal cookbook *Nourishing Traditions*, modern farming, food storage, and food production methods damage both the quality of the food supply and the people who consume it. Fallon claims that only by adopting our ancestors' farming and food preparation methods can we meet our nutritional requirements and enjoy perfect health. Her book documents the many ways in which traditional methods improve the digestibility of grains and other foods.

Soaking removes phytic acid, an organic acid in untreated grain which combines with calcium, magnesium, copper, iron, and zinc in the intestinal tract, blocking their absorption. According to Fallon, phytic acid is the reason why a modern diet high in whole grains can lead to serious mineral deficiencies and bone loss. Overnight soaking in warm water destroys phytates, neutralizes the enzyme inhibitors present in all grains, increases the production of beneficial enzymes, breaks down gluten (a difficult-to-digest protein found in most grains), and makes grains less likely to cause allergic reactions.

Whole rice and millet contain fewer phytates than other grains, and they are gluten-free, which makes them easier to digest even without presoaking. However, these grains should be cooked very slowly over low heat, preferably in homemade broth or stock, to facilitate digestion. Microwave ovens and pressure cookers damage the fats and proteins in grains and are not recommended.

Traditional Porridge

To make a traditional porridge, soak 1 cup cracked, rolled, or coarsely ground oats, rice, kamut, spelt, rye, or other grain in 1 cup filtered water plus 2 tablespoons whey, yogurt, kefir, or buttermilk for seven to twenty-four hours. Those with severe milk sensitivities or a lactose intolerance can substitute lemon juice for the whey, yogurt, kefir, or buttermilk. Teff, amaranth, and rye benefit from a twenty-four-hour soaking, and rye may need additional water for complete hydration.

In traditional cultures, corn or maize was always soaked in lime water. This process releases vitamin B_3, which is otherwise unavailable, and it improves the amino acid quality of proteins in the corn's germ. To make lime water, place 1 inch of dolomite powder (sold as a supplement in health food stores) in a 2-quart glass jar. Fill the jar with filtered water, cover tightly, shake well, and let stand overnight. The resulting lime water does not require refrigeration. To use, pour off what you need without disturbing the settled powder. To replenish the jar, add filtered water, cover, and shake well. Always soak grits, cornmeal, and coarsely ground corn in lime water before cooking.

Bring 1 cup filtered water to a boil. Add the soaked grain and ½ teaspoon sea salt. Reduce heat, cover, and simmer for several minutes, stirring occasionally. Soaking shortens cooking time considerably, and most porridge is thick and fully cooked in five to ten minutes.

Germination

The process of germination or sprouting changes grains into living foods that are rich in vitamins, trace minerals, the carbohydrate-digesting enzyme amylase, amino acids, and other nutrients. Sprouting increases a grain's vitamin K content by as much as twenty-five times and its carotene by up to twelve times. B-complex vitamins such as pantothenic acid typically increase by up to 200 percent, vitamin B_{12} by over 500 percent, pyridoxine by 600 percent, and riboflavin by nearly 150 percent during sprouting.

To sprout, soak ½ to 1 cup organically grown grain (rice is the only grain for which this method is not recommended) in a wide-mouth quart jar. Fill the jar with water and soak the grain for seven to twelve hours or overnight. For increased mineral content, add a pinch of powdered or liquid kelp to the soak water.

Health food stores sell plastic sprouting lids for wide-mouth quart jars, or you can fashion a sprouting lid with cheesecloth and a rubber band. Sprouting lid in place, drain the jar well, then lay it on its side in a warm place away from direct sunlight. Ideal sprouting temperatures are between 70 and 80 degrees Fahrenheit.

After twenty-four to thirty-six hours, you will see small white roots emerge from the grain. If you don't see this growth on almost every seed by the second day, your grain is not viable and should be discarded. Sprouting grain can be used in any recipe calling for grain. Use the grain's presprouting measurement and reduce the amount of liquid the recipe calls for. Sprouting grain can be ground or pureed in a food processor and used in place of or in addition to flour in breads and baked goods. At first, add small amounts of sprouted grain to familiar recipes, then later, you can experiment.

Another way to improve the digestibility of breads and baked goods is with sourdough fermentation. This slow-rise method, used around the world until baker's yeast became popular, breaks down phytates and enzyme inhibitors in flour while increasing the digestibility and nutritional content of grains. Most health food stores sell naturally fermented breads; look for labels that say "yeast-free" or "sourdough." Make your own with the help of a commercial sourdough starter, or follow the directions in *Nourishing Traditions* or bread-making cookbooks.

Sprouted Grain Casserole

Soaked, sprouted grains can be used in side dishes and casseroles. Fallon's basic recipe combines 2 cups sprouting grain with 3 cups beef or chicken stock. Bring to a boil and skim. Add 1 teaspoon sea salt and ½ teaspoon each dried thyme, rosemary, and crushed green peppercorns. Boil vigorously until the liquid is reduced to the level of the grain. Transfer to a 250-degree Fahrenheit oven, cover, and bake for approximately four hours, or until the grain is tender.

Soaking Nuts

Nuts have a well-deserved reputation for being difficult to digest. Like grains and seeds, they contain enzyme inhibitors that can interfere with digestion, causing discomfort or a heavy feeling in the stomach or abdomen.

To remove these enzyme inhibitors, add 2 teaspoons salt to 4 cups raw, shelled nuts, cover with filtered water, and soak eight to twelve hours. Cashews, which are roasted during harvesting, should be soaked for no more than six hours.

Drain the soaked nuts in a colander, then place them in a food dehydrator according to the manufacturer's instructions, or spread them on a stainless steel baking pan left in a barely warm oven (less than 150 degrees Fahrenheit) for twelve to twenty-four hours. Turn the nuts occasionally, until they are completely dry and crisp. Store in a tightly sealed container in the refrigerator.

FATS AND OILS

Saturated fats, unsaturated fats, hydrogenated fats, trans-fatty acids, good cholesterol, bad cholesterol, high-fat diets, low-fat diets, artificial fats, essential fats—the experts' claims about fats in the diet are so contradictory they make the head spin.

A detailed examination of fats, their chemistry, and their action in the body is beyond the scope of this book, so here are some simple guidelines that will help you recognize the fats you need while avoiding those that cause harm.

Essential fatty acids or EFAs are the building blocks of fats. There are two main essential fats: linoleic acid (LA, or omega-6 polyunsaturated fatty acid) and alpha-linoleic acid (LNA, or omega-3 superunsaturated fatty acid). Gamma linoleic acid (GLA), which belongs to the first group, is a key regulator of T-lymphocyte function in the body.

EFA deficiencies cause circulatory problems and may contribute to cancer as well as skin diseases, liver and kidney problems, slow or incomplete wound healing, weight problems, behavior changes, joint pain, dry eyes, vision problems, a lack of coordination, learning disabilities, fluid retention, skin dryness, splitting nails, hangnails, fibromyalgia, heart disease, pulmonary disorders, hormone imbalances, diabetes, skin eruptions similar to eczema, hair loss, glandular problems, dehydration, susceptibility to infections, sterility in males, miscarriage in females, tingling sensations in the legs and arms, and even death. All but the last condition can be reversed by adding the proper balance of EFAs to the diet.

For most adults, between 1 and 2 tablespoons of the right fats and oils provide adequate levels of EFAs. Sunflower, safflower, soybean, and corn oils are rich in omega-6, while fish, flaxseed, and walnut oils are rich in omega-3. According to EFA researcher Udo Erasmus, author of the book *Fats That Heal, Fats That Kill,* the ideal ratio of omega-6 to omega-3 in human nutrition is 2 to 1 or 3 to 1. Most traditional diets fall within this range, but modern diets that emphasize safflower and corn oils are so unbalanced, with ratios of up to 20 to 1, are seriously deficient in omega-3.

The oils that nourished healthy populations for thousands of years are butter and other animal fats, coconut oil, palm oil, sesame seed oil, olive oil, fish, and fish oils.

The Saturated/Unsaturated/TFA Debate

Saturated fats are usually solid at room temperature, which distinguishes them from unsaturated fats, which are liquid. The two dietary sources of naturally saturated fats are animal fats, which are found in beef, pork, poultry, butter, and cheese; and tropical oils, including coconut, palm, and palm kernel oils.

These fats, as everyone knows, can be dangerous to eat. They clog arteries, disrupt the immune system, and do all kinds of damage. Or do they?

That depends. Beef tallow that is repeatedly used for deep-fat frying in fast-food restaurants (think of everyone's favorite, french fries) is so carcinogenic that it can't be recycled as a food for humans. Instead, it is sent to rendering plants and sold as a pet food ingredient.

At the same time, saturated fats are an integral part of traditional cuisines that have kept people healthy for thousands of years. Butter, described on page 76, is one example; coconut oil is another. According to Mary G. Enig, Ph.D., a Weston A. Price

Foundation associate and author of the book *Know Your Fats: Understanding the Nutrition of Fats, Oils, and Cholesterol*, coconut oil's bad reputation stems from an incorrect interpretation of results obtained when animals were fed coconut oil that was purposely altered by hydrogenation to remove its essential fatty acids. The animals became deficient in EFAs, and their serum cholesterol levels increased.

The food industry soon replaced coconut oil with hydrogenated or partially hydrogenated monounsaturated and polyunsaturated oils such as canola and soybean. However, unsaturated vegetable oils spoil easily, and when heated or hydrogenated, their unsaturated fatty acids deform from a natural, curved shape to an unnatural, jointed shape called a trans-configuration. This shape is the signature of trans-fatty acids or TFAs.

Research has shown that these new fats are more dangerous than the coconut and palm oils they replaced. In November 1999, the FDA requested that manufacturers include trans fats on food product labels because of their link to heart disease and death. Any product containing hydrogenated or partially hydrogenated oil is a significant source of TFAs.

After news about trans-fatty acids adversely affected margarine sales, food processors developed a new type of margarine that is free of TFAs. Suddenly, trans-fatty-acid-free margarine became a health food.

Don't buy the hype, says Bruce West, D.C., whose *Health Alert* newsletter emphasizes whole-food nutrition. "While these liquid plastics may lower your cholesterol level slightly," he warns, "they also wreak havoc on the core of your health, including your cell membranes." According to West, compromising the health of every cell in the body to achieve an insignificant drop in cholesterol levels is a dangerous mistake.

Cooking with Oils

The best oils for salads and EFA supplementation are far too fragile to cook with. Flax, evening primrose, black currant, and borage seed oils break down even at low heat.

Unrefined, cold-pressed olive, sunflower, safflower, sesame, walnut, corn, soy, and pumpkin seed oils tolerate some heat before they begin to break down. Considered medium-heat cooking oils, they are best for light sautéeing and sauces and should not be heated above 320 degrees Fahrenheit (160 degrees Celsius). Peanut oil, which belongs to this category if unrefined, remains a questionable oil even if organically produced because it is often contaminated with aflatoxin, a carcinogenic fungus. Peanuts are legumes rather than nuts. If conventionally grown, they are treated with so many pesticides and fungicides that typical peanuts contain traces of 186 different chemicals. In addition, allergic reactions to peanuts can be fatal. For these reasons, peanut oil is best approached with caution.

Conditioned or semi-refined canola, corn, soy, sunflower, grapeseed, safflower, and sesame oils have a milder flavor than these same oils do when unrefined, and they withstand the higher heat of baking, stir-frying, and sautéeing at temperatures up to 375 degrees Fahrenheit (190 degrees Celsius). However, the chemical treatment of unsaturated vegetable oils strips them of fragile nutrients and creates trans-fatty acids.

Bland-tasting, highly refined avocado, high-oleic sunflower, high-oleic safflower, peanut, almond, rice bran, apricot kernel, and sesame oils begin smoking at temperatures between 410 and 520 degrees Fahrenheit. In their natural state, these oils burn at low temperatures, but the chemical processing that removes their nutrients makes them suitable for searing, browning, deep-fat frying, and pan frying. It also makes them dangerous, for these are the oils most likely to cause heart disease, cancer, immune dysfunction, sterility, learning problems, growth problems, and osteoporosis.

According to William Campbell Douglass, M.D., in the April 1998 edition of his *Second Opinion* newsletter, coconut oil is an important oil for cooking because it protects against thyroid gland and immune system suppression, enables one to maintain a normal weight without effort, provides important nutrition to the brain, contains important nutrients such as butyric acid, helps maintain healthy fat and cholesterol levels in the blood, and has antihistamine, antidiabetic, anticancer, and anti-infective properties. For importers of unrefined, organic coconut oil, see the Resources.

Slow cooking over gentle heat is far less damaging to foods than deep-fat frying, pressure cooking, and high-temperature grilling. Whenever possible, heat, bake, or roast foods at low rather than high heat, cook eggs in their shell or poach instead of frying them, and avoid fried, deep-fat fried, burned, and pressure-canned foods.

The Truth about Butter

Despite what you've heard, butter is one of the healthiest fats you can consume. It contains considerable amounts of unsaturated fatty acids and is an excellent source of fat-soluble vitamins. Butter's saturated fat molecules are extremely short, making them easy for the body to digest and burn as fuel. Its short-chain fatty acids are a good food for the liver; in addition, they help intestinal flora stay healthy, have antiviral, antifungal, antibacterial, and antitumor properties, and help lower cholesterol. In addition, butter withstands the heat of cooking far better than any unprocessed vegetable oil. It is the most versatile all-purpose fat for cooking.

There is no denying that butter is high in calories. It is also 100 percent fat, so proponents of low-fat diets have nothing good to say about it. However, despite a widespread belief to the contrary, no medical study has ever established a link between butter and heart disease. Whenever butter is added to the diets of laboratory animals, they gain weight, but they never develop arterial plaque or any type of circulatory problem.

The main cause of butter's bad reputation is advertising. Margarine has been promoted as the healthier spread for so long that most Americans believe it's true. On the contrary, research has shown that margarine and shortening, both of which contain hydrogenated vegetable oils, are highly detrimental to one's health. Other harmful oils are chemically extracted vegetable oils, which include all of the popular, inexpensive oils sold in supermarkets. Switching from margarine, vegetable shortening, and mass-produced vegetable oil to organically grown butter is one of the best things you can do for your health.

EFA Oil and "Better Butter"

To make an EFA-oil blend, combine two parts flaxseed oil with one part sesame, almond, pumpkin seed, coconut, or other seed or nut oil. Alternatively, buy an EFA blend. Oils should be cold-pressed, organically grown, and as fresh as possible. This oil blend, which should not be heated, can be added to salads and other foods.

To make a soft spread with additional health benefits, combine 1 cup unrefined EFA-rich oil with 1 pound softened butter and mix in a food processor, blender, hand mixer, or by hand until combined.

If available, use raw butter from healthy cattle. Raw butter contains enzymes and other nutrients that are destroyed by pasteurization. Alternatively, you can make your own butter from piima cream (see Resources).

If desired, add 1 teaspoon unrefined sea salt.

Store in an airtight container and refrigerate. As this Better Butter should not be heated, add it to food just before serving. One to 2 tablespoons per day provide a well-balanced blend of essential fatty acids.

CHOLESTEROL MYTHS

Cholesterol is a white, waxy, fatlike substance manufactured by the liver that is essential to life. It is present in the blood and most tissues, especially those of the nervous system, and it is an important fuel for the brain and nerves. Cholesterol and its esters are important constituents of cell membranes throughout the body and the precursors of many steroid hormones and bile salts.

For decades, high cholesterol levels have been associated with arterial blockage, circulatory impairment, and other symptoms of heart disease. Plants do not contain cholesterol, but animal foods do, and patients with high blood pressure are warned to reduce their intake of eggs, meat, and saturated fat. Doing so is supposed to reduce both blood cholesterol levels and the risk of having a heart attack.

The only thing wrong with this theory is that it doesn't work. William Castelli, director of the world's largest heart research project, the Framingham Heart Study, reported in the *Archives of Internal Medicine* in 1992 that the more saturated fat, cholesterol, and calories his study's participants ate, the lower their serum cholesterol. "We found that people who ate the most cholesterol, ate the most saturated fat, and ate the most calories weighed the least and were the most physically active," he said.

Renowned heart surgeon Michael De Bakey, M.D., found that in 1,700 patients with clogged blood vessels, an analysis of cholesterol levels "revealed no definite correlation between serum cholesterol levels and the nature and extent of the atherosclerotic disease."

According to Russell L. Smith, Ph.D., author of an authoritative study on coronary heart disease, "The relevant literature on coronary heart disease is permeated with fraudulent material that is designed to convert negative evidence into positive evidence with respect to the lipid [saturated fat] hypothesis."

George Mann, M.D., an acclaimed medical researcher, explains that the discredited cholesterol theory is kept alive by those who profit from it financially. "The hypothesis continues to be exploited by scientists, fund-raising enterprises, food companies, and even government agencies," he wrote. "The public is being deceived by the greatest health scam of the century."

In October 1997, the British medical journal *The Lancet* published research showing that in elderly patients, those with the highest cholesterol levels lived the longest. Serum cholesterol levels below 200 combined with low albumin levels (below 4) in those over age seventy corresponded to an increased risk of degenerating health and death.

Total cholesterol levels are now known to have little correlation to circulatory health. Rather, HDL ("good" cholesterol) and its ratio to total cholesterol is important. In addition, a person's total cholesterol level is a useful marker for comparing triglyceride levels. For good health, triglyceride levels should not exceed total cholesterol.

Unfortunately, Americans have increasingly high triglyceride levels, which are often caused by an excessive consumption of carbohydrates. Most patients with high triglyceride levels can lower them quickly by reducing or eliminating bread, grains, and sugars.

THE MILK DEBATE

Americans think of milk as one of the safest, most nutritious, and necessary foods for infants, children, and adults. But a growing number of physicians disagree, including Frank Oski, M.D., who was head of the Pediatrics Department of New York University when he wrote *Don't Drink Your Milk!* According to Dr. Oski, 25 percent of children fed cow's milk before age six will develop one or more allergies from it. This is, he explains, because cow's milk proteins neutralize hydrochloric acid in the stomach, making the digestive system work harder to produce enough HCl to digest food. Over time, incomplete digestion allows protein molecules to become absorbed when only partially broken down, disrupting the normal function of tissues and organs.

Casein, the principal protein in cow's milk, is well utilized by calves, but humans find it difficult to digest. Many pediatricians link repeated ear infections, colds, and coughs in children to bacteria-breeding mucus created throughout the body by poorly digested casein from dairy products. As soon as their patients stop consuming milk, ice cream, cottage cheese, and other milk products, ear infections disappear.

The consumption of dairy products has been linked to other illnesses, such as diabetes. Researchers at the National Institute of Diabetes and Digestive and Kidney Diseases in Phoenix, Arizona, studied 720 Pima Indians, a group with a high prevalence of non-insulin dependent diabetes mellitus (NIDDM), and found that those who were exclusively breast-fed had significantly lower rates of NIDDM than those who received infant formulas. In separate studies, babies who were breast-fed exclusively for the first two months of life had a far lower rate of NIDDM than those who received cow's milk formulas instead of or in addition to breast milk. Over eighty studies published in the 1990s implicate cow's milk consumption in juvenile-onset diabetes, including a Finnish study in which 100 percent of 172 newly diagnosed juvenile diabetes patients had very high levels of antibodies to cow's milk.

The research of Kurt A. Oster, M.D., shows that homogenization may be a culprit in allergies and other illnesses associated with milk consumption, including heart disease, which is not an affliction unique to old age. An estimated 10,000 children die of heart attacks every year on playgrounds in the United States and Canada. Cow's milk contains large fat molecules that effectively feed baby calves but pass through the digestive tracts of humans. However, homogenization breaks down fat particles to such a small size that virtually all of the fat is absorbed by body tissues not normally exposed to it. In addition, milk fat contains an enzyme which is not normally available to the human body but which is freed by homogenization. When the enzyme escapes digestion, it is transported by fat globules through the intestinal wall and into the circulatory system. Dr. Oster and other researchers believe that by replacing normal heart tissue components, this enzyme triggers atherosclerosis. This does not occur when milk is left in its natural state without being homogenized.

Cow's milk and dairy products made from it have been blamed for diarrhea, cramps, constipation, gastrointestinal bleeding, iron-deficiency anemia, skin rashes, atherosclerosis, acne, recurrent ear infections, bronchitis, dental decay, respiratory problems, asthma, hay fever allergies, rheumatoid arthritis, and a host of other problems in humans of all ages. Much of the evidence is anecdotal, but eliminating pasteurized, homogenized cow's milk from the diet has alleviated so many symptoms in children and adults that this simple strategy has become increasingly popular.

According to Sally Fallon, what passes for milk in America today could not keep a calf healthy and is bad for humans, as well. In addition to being contaminated with growth hormone and antibiotic residues, milk from cows that are fed unnatural feeds such as soy and cottonseed meal is deficient in essential fatty acids and fat-soluble vitamins. Pasteurization destroys enzymes, diminishes vitamin content, denatures protein, alters vitamin B_{12}, destroys vitamin B_6, kills beneficial bacteria, and promotes harmful bacteria. Ultrapasteurization, which involves higher temperatures and longer processing, is even more damaging. Raw milk sours naturally, but pasteurized milk only rots and becomes putrid.

The production of low-fat and skim milk is a convenient way for the dairy industry to sell unwanted milk left over after butterfat is removed. Both are deficient in natural vitamins, fats, and other nutrients. Powdered skim milk, which contains oxidized cholesterol and neurotoxins, is added to low-fat (1 and 2 percent) milk. This potentially harmful ingredient, which is often labeled nonfat milk solids, is added to most brands of yogurt, sour cream, kefir, cream cheese, and cottage cheese. Synthetic vitamin D, which is difficult to digest and absorb, is added to liquid milk, various chemicals are added to dairy products, and most butter is dyed yellow. Unprocessed whole milk and butter from healthy, organically raised, grass-fed cattle is superior in every way, but its sale is illegal in most states.

Fallon created an organization called A Campaign for Real Milk (see Resources) to educate Americans about real milk, develop a legal fund to bring a court case to the Supreme Court to once again make real milk legal in all states, and publish a list of real milk suppliers throughout the United States.

Raw milk cheeses are sold in several states (some of the world's finest are imported from France), and many Americans have friendly relations with local dairy cows or goats which keep them supplied with the real thing. Frances Pottenger, M.D., a leading medical researcher in the 1930s and '40s, measured the growth and health of infants fed infant formula, their own mothers' milk, boiled cow's milk, and whole, raw, cow's milk. The healthiest children were fed by healthy mothers who ate a well-balanced diet of whole foods, but infants fed raw cow's milk developed stronger bones and were healthier than infants breast-fed by mothers who ate an inferior diet.

Dairy products were used by only a few traditional cultures around the world, but in all of those cases, the dairy products that kept people healthy were raw, organically grown, unpasteurized, and unhomogenized. Fortunately, unhomogenized milk that is pasteurized but not ultrapasteurized is available in many health food stores. It can be used to make yogurt, kefir, and piima (see Resources) as well as dairy products like cream cheese, whey, butter, and buttermilk. These home-prepared foods, which are easy to make, are superior in every way to the dairy products in American markets.

CHAPTER FOUR

Nutritional Supplements

FOOD IS IMPORTANT, BUT EVEN the ideal diet may need assistance. Between stress, environmental pollution, a nutritionally deficient food supply, and our tendency to eat on the run, most of us need more nutrients than our diets provide.

The following supplements correct nutritional deficiencies as well as the damage caused by prior nutritional imbalances. As a result, they help prevent, improve, reverse, and cure many conditions that cause discomfort, such as respiratory problems, digestive disorders, arthritis, slow-healing wounds, sports injuries, and all types of chronic disorders, including those considered incurable by orthodox physicians.

All the products described here are well tolerated by most users. Anyone taking a product for the first time should exercise common sense, for individual allergic reactions are always possible. First-time users, especially those with a history of allergies, should take the smallest recommended amount and watch for unusual symptoms. It is easy to check for allergic reactions with the pulse test (see pages 59 to 60), four-day rotation diet (see pages 58 to 59), or by keeping a journal and noting health changes as they occur.

Nutritional deficiencies often develop slowly, and it takes time to reverse them as well. Improvement may be noticeable within a few days or weeks, but best results usually follow after months or years of improved nutrition.

Health food stores, supermarkets, and pharmacies are full of "natural" products promising a quick fix for every imaginable disorder. However, many such products aren't natural at all. This chapter will help you make sense of the claims in ads and on package labels.

HYDROCHLORIC ACID

The high-sugar, low-fiber, nutrient-depleted American diet sustains life; we'd all be dead if it didn't. The fact that it doesn't enhance health isn't obvious, though, or more people would stop eating it. Dietary habits are set in youth, when the body has an abundance of enzymes and gastric juices that help compensate for nutritional deficiencies.

Things change in middle age, which is when most chronic illnesses manifest themselves. One reason is that as the body ages, it produces less hydrochloric acid (HCl), which leads to indigestion and an inability to absorb nutrients. Hydrochloric acid is a powerful chemical that breaks down food fibers, digests proteins, and destroys harmful bacteria. It's an important factor in preventing disease. Most people believe that their indigestion or discomfort is due to too much stomach acid, but it is generally caused when the body produces less. When people take antacids, the further suppress their stomach's ability to generate hydrochloric acid, which makes the problem worse. An insufficient supply of hydrochloric acid interferes with digestion and leaves one more vulnerable to bacterial, viral, or microbial infections.

Jonathan V. Wright, M.D., a leading expert on nutrition and health, has found that gastric hypochlorhydria (insufficient stomach acid), which results in incomplete protein digestion, a major cause of allergies, brittle nails, thinning hair, and skin problems, is extremely common in those over forty. Adequate levels of hydrochloric acid are required for the absorption of amino acids, minerals, and vitamins, especially vitamin B_{12}, iron, zinc, and calcium. Many illnesses are associated with low stomach acidity, including osteoporosis, rheumatoid arthritis, and lupus erythematosus.

Although orthodox medicine rejects the use of digestive supplements, Dr. Wright has found that they often improve a patient's overall health as well as specific symptoms, such as inflammation and pain. He cautions against using hydrochloric acid by itself (it works better in combination with pepsin) or in tablets because powdered HCl in capsules works more efficiently. If any discomfort such as pain, burning, or additional gas is experienced after taking HCl/pepsin supplements, he suggests diluting the powder in water and taking very small amounts, increasing the quantity to standard doses over a period of weeks.

Although there are medical tests that check for insufficient HCl levels, it is easy to test for this condition at home. If a tablespoon of cider vinegar or lemon juice taken with dinner causes discomfort, your HCl levels are probably high or normal. If vinegar or lemon juice seems to relieve after-dinner discomfort, your HCl level is probably low. Try taking an HCl supplement and experiment with the recommended label dosage, increasing it as needed. Another simple way to test HCl levels is called the beet juice test: Drink ½ cup beet juice daily for three days. If your urine turns red, this may be a general indication that HCl and enzymes, including pepsin, may be needed to improve your digestion and the assimilation of nutrients.

Research conducted in the 1940s showed that the amount of HCl needed to fully acidify an average size dinner to a pH of 1.8 to 2.2 is the amount contained in thirty 650-milligram capsules of betaine hydrochloride. Dr. Wright has observed that when HCl levels are insufficient, the average adult needs five to seven 650-milligram capsules per meal. The dosage recommended on most product labels, which is substantially less than this, may be ineffective.

Hydrochloric acid, and digestive supplements that contain it, should not be taken on an empty stomach. They are not recommended for ulcer patients or for the few who (unlike most Americans) truly do have excessive stomach acid.

DIGESTIVE ENZYMES

Unless you eat almost everything raw, your food is organically grown on farmland rich in minerals, and you've enjoyed perfect health for decades, your digestion probably needs assistance.

Enzymes are proteins that, in small amounts, speed the rate of biological reactions. Unstable and easily inactivated by heat and certain chemicals, enzymes are produced within living cells to perform specific biochemical reactions. Nearly every raw food carries within it the enzymes necessary for its digestion, but cooking inactivates enzymes and the body must work hard to replace them in order for food to be broken down and assimilated.

Enzyme supplements derived from pineapples, figs, papayas, fungi, bacteria, animals, and other sources replace at least some of the enzymes killed by the cooking and processing of food. They can be taken with raw foods, too, especially by those who are recovering from an illness, have been treated with antibiotics, or are experiencing any digestive difficulty. Enzyme supplements (see Resources) have impressive records of safety and health improvement.

Plant-derived enzymes include protease, which digests protein; lipase, an upper digestive-tract enzyme that breaks down fats or lipids; and amylase, a saliva enzyme that digests starch or carbohydrates. Proteases, or proteolytic enzymes, include many different enzymes, each of which breaks down a specific amino acid found in protein. For example, trypsin interacts with the amino acids arginine and lysine, and chymotrypsin breaks down tyrosine, tryptophan, and phenylalanine. Lipases, or lipolytic enzymes, digest lipids, including phospholipids such as lecithin, sterols such as cholesterol, and triglycerides, which are oils and fats. Amylases, or amylytic enzymes, interact with carbohydrates, including lactose, a sugar in milk and other dairy products; fructose, a simple sugar found in honey and sweet fruits; starches, which occur in almost all plant foods, especially grains; and sucrose, the disaccharide found in cane sugar and beet sugar, which contains fructose and glucose. The human body does not produce cellulase, which digests cellulose, the fiber or roughage found in plants.

Coenzymes are nonprotein substances that combine with protein to form a complete enzyme. Most of the coenzymes important in human nutrition are produced from vitamins or are themselves vitamins. Lipoic acid, which was once thought to be a member of the B-vitamin complex, and coenzyme Q10, which resembles vitamin E, are popular supplements because they help prevent and treat chronic illnesses. For example, lipoic acid, which is abundant in red meat, is a powerful antioxidant that removes toxins from the body, helps prevent cataracts, increases immune function, and improves the health of nerves.

Coenzyme Q10, another important antioxidant, has been used to treat cancer, improve respiratory function, heal ulcers, prevent allergies, and improve heart health. Mackerel, salmon, and sardines are the leading food sources of coenzyme Q10. Like food enzymes, coenzymes deteriorate at temperatures above approximately 115 degrees Fahrenheit. Antioxidant enzymes, found in fresh sprouts, convert potentially damaging free radicals to harmless oxygen and water. The best known antioxidant enzymes are superoxide dismutase (SOD), catalase, glutathione peroxidase, and methionine reductase.

Pancreatic enzymes are usually derived from the pancreas of cattle. Pancreatin works only in the small intestine. Taken with food, it assists in the digestion of protein, fats, and carbohydrates, and it can prevent adverse food reactions. Taken on an empty stomach, it reduces inflammation and pain throughout the body and helps eliminate intestinal parasites by literally digesting them.

Most digestive enzyme products contain some combination of protease, amylase, and lipase. Some brands include hydrochloric acid, pepsin, ox bile, pancreatic substances, papain from papaya, cellulose enzymes, bromelain from pineapple, and others. Digestive enzymes are sold as powders to sprinkle on food or as tablets or capsules. There are dozens on the market, including vegetarian formulas, special blends, and products for dogs and cats. Whenever you eat cooked or processed food, especially as you grow older, consider taking an enzyme supplement.

One single-ingredient, special-purpose enzyme supplement makes beans, legumes, and soybean products easier to digest, and helps prevent flatulence. Another contains lactase, the enzyme that digests milk sugar. Beano (for beans) and Lactaid (for milk) were the first of these products; now several brands make bean and dairy dishes easier to digest.

SYSTEMIC ORAL ENZYME THERAPY

Enzyme therapy does not just refer to supplements taken with food. Some digestive enzymes taken between meals, on an empty stomach, improve health throughout the body. For example, the enzyme bromelain has been shown to reduce swelling and bruising from trauma injuries, improve circulation while reducing inflammation and clotting in those with heart disease, speed wound healing, relax cramping muscles during menstruation, relieve chronic pain, reduce sinus congestion and inflammation, alleviate tendinitis, reduce skin irritation associated with varicose veins, and reverse many of the effects of scleroderma, an autoimmune disease that causes severe hardening and thickening of the skin and connective tissue. Papain has anti-inflammatory and wound-healing properties. Other digestive enzymes reduce inflammation, improve immune function, and stimulate the digestion of bacteria, toxins, and partly digested proteins, cleansing the lymph and blood of problem-causing particles.

Some health care practitioners have discovered that digestive enzymes taken at night, several hours after dinner, relieve food sensitivities, hay fever allergies, and insomnia caused by reactions to food.

The Aspirin Alternative by Michael Loes, M.D., describes the many ways in which systemic oral enzyme therapy can be used in place of nonsteroidal anti-inflammatory drugs (NSAIDs). Dr. Loes recommends the German product Wobenzym N, which contains pancreatin, trypsin, chymotrypsin, bromelain, papain, and rutosid, but other enzyme products have produced similar results.

In systemic oral enzyme therapy, the maintenance dose for adults is three to five Wobenzym N tablets forty-five minutes before meals three times daily. Patients with serious illnesses or infections may need up to thirty tablets per day until symptoms improve. This therapy has helped cure, reverse, or improve osteoarthritis, rheumatoid arthritis, systemic lupus erythematosus, ankylosing spondylitis, tooth infections, oral surgery, vascular surgery, trauma injuries, bone fractures, knee surgery, sports injuries, heart disease, acute and chronic bronchitis, sinusitis, prostatitis, cystitis, lower urinary tract infections, pelvic inflammatory disease, herpes zoster (shingles), ulcerative colitis, Crohn's disease, pancreatitis, chlamydia, multiple sclerosis, tinnitus, and fibrocystic breast disease. In most cases, patients improved dramatically or made a complete recovery. European athletes on systemic oral enzyme therapy recovered quickly from sports injuries, and some made spectacular comebacks during the Olympics and other events. In the German studies cited by Dr. Loes, some patients received conventional drugs such as antibiotics, and their infections cleared more rapidly than expected. The therapy also prevented high-risk patients from developing serious illnesses, such as children at risk of developing juvenile diabetes.

Systemic oral enzyme therapy is safe, inexpensive, easy to follow, and effective. When taking enzymes between meals, it is important to use products that do not contain hydrochloric acid (HCl), as that digestive aid should not be taken on an empty stomach except when recommended for such use.

BENEFICIAL BACTERIA

For information about acidophilus and other probiotic supplements, see the Resources.

VITAMINS

Vitamins are substances required in small amounts for healthy growth and development. Because they cannot be synthesized in the body, they are essential constituents of the diet. Vitamins are divided into two groups according to whether they are soluble in water or fat. The water-soluble group includes the vitamin B complex, vitamin C, and bioflavonoids, which are sometimes called vitamin P. The fat-soluble vitamins are A, D, E, and K, all of which are stored in the body, and essential fatty acids, which are sometimes called vitamin F. Lack of sufficient quantities of any of these vitamins or their close relatives manifests as a deficiency disease or some form of impaired health.

Many physicians believe that vitamin supplements are both a waste of money and potentially harmful. Others, who appreciate the nutritional shortcomings of America's food supply, believe they are essential to good health. Of those who recommend supplements, some favor large doses of synthetic vitamins, while others recommend small doses of vitamins derived from whole foods. Making sense of the vitamin industry can be a daunting task.

Vitamin A, a fat-soluble nutrient, is essential for the maintenance of soft mucous tissues, normal growth, and healthy eyes. Deficiencies cause stunted growth, night blindness, and other vision disorders. Beta carotene in foods such as carrots and yams converts to vitamin A in the human body, and foods such as deep-sea fish oils are rich in this nutrient.

The B-complex vitamins (thiamine, niacin, riboflavin, biotin, folic acid, pantothenic acid, and others) are vital to the health of the nervous system, and deficiencies in this group can manifest as symptoms anywhere in the body, most often in the mouth, eyes, and reproductive organs. These are among the most fragile and heat-sensitive vitamins. Like vitamin C, they are water-soluble and are not stored in the body. Liver and other organ meats, fish, poultry, brewer's yeast, eggs, beans, peas, dark green leafy vegetables, whole grains, and dairy products are rich sources of B-complex vitamins.

Vitamin C, by far the world's most popular vitamin, is an antioxidant needed for tissue growth and repair, adrenal gland function, and healthy gums. In addition to protecting the body from the harmful effects of environmental toxins and stress, it improves immunity, speeds wound healing, protects against infection, and helps prevent cancer, harmful blood clotting, and bruising. It is found in green vegetables, chili peppers, berries, and citrus fruit.

There are a thousand or more bioflavonoids, which usually occur in combination with vitamin C in leaves, bark, rinds, flowers, and seeds. While bioflavonoids often act as coloring pigments in plants, their more important function for human nutrition appears to be their synergistic partnership with vitamin C. Citrus fruits are high in hesperidin and eriocitrin, buckwheat is rich in rutin, and other sprouts are rich in quercetin, to name four of the most familiar bioflavonoids.

Vitamin D is called the sunshine vitamin because exposure to sunlight manufactures it in the body. Vitamin D, which is also supplied by foods such as fatty fish, shellfish, lard, free-range chicken egg yokes, and organ meats, is necessary for calcium and phosphorus absorption and utilization. In children, it is essential for normal skeletal growth and the development of teeth and bones; in adults, it helps prevent and treat osteoporosis and improves immunity. Research on the elderly has shown that high blood levels of vitamin D and normal thyroid function are the strongest markers of health and longevity. Recent findings indicate that vitamin D may protect against cancer, diabetes, cataracts, infertility, premenstrual syndrome (PMS), chronic fatigue, seasonal affective disorder (SAD), and other illnesses.

While too much sun exposure can be harmful, today's widespread use of sunscreens and protective clothing has produced a nationwide vitamin D deficiency.

Exposing the arms, legs, and face to summer sunlight for ten to twenty minutes a day at least three days per week is widely reported to produce significant amounts of vitamin D. However, this exposure provides only 200 to 400 international units (IU) of vitamin D at a time and only during summer months in the middle of the day. In order to achieve optimal levels of vitamin D, 85 percent of the body needs exposure to the midday sun, between 10 A.M. and 2 P.M. Light-skinned people need ten to twenty minutes of exposure while dark-skinned people need one and a half to two hours.

Another way to raise vitamin D levels is with supplements, but it is impossible to prescribe a specific dose because the amount of vitamin D that brings one person to optimum health may be toxic (or insufficient) for someone else. Vitamin D researcher and clinical nutritionist Krispin Sullivan recommends using a blood test to diagnose a vitamin D deficiency and monitor vitamin D levels during supplementation. For information about vitamin D blood tests and appropriate supplementation, see the Resources.

Because of their interdependency, vitamin D, calcium, and magnesium should be taken together.

Vitamin E is essential during every phase of life, including gestation. Mothers with high vitamin E levels tend to have stronger, healthier babies and easier birthings than those with low levels. Vitamin E speeds the healing of wounds and burns, improves the assimilation and distribution of nutrients throughout the body, keeps the heart healthy, slows the symptoms of aging, improves the skin and hair, and boosts resistance to disease. Food sources of vitamin E include vegetable oils, nuts, dark green, leafy vegetables, organ meats, seafood, eggs, and avocados. People with heart disease, athletes, and those under stress benefit from supplemental vitamin E.

Vitamin K regulates blood clotting and other clotting factors; it is also essential for kidney function and bone metabolism. Food sources include beef liver, cheese, oats, cabbage, turnip greens, and other dark green, leafy vegetables.

Natural versus Synthetic

In any discussion of supplements, it's necessary to examine the differences between vitamins and other nutrients found in food and their synthetic counterparts. Nobel Prizes have been awarded for vitamin synthesis; the scientific community regards synthetics as identical to natural nutrients; and the low cost of synthetic supplements makes them affordable to all.

But are synthetic and natural nutrients really the same? Molecular structures can match in two dimensions without being identical. A complex three-dimensional shape that doesn't exactly match its model will never behave exactly like the original. Living bodies can tell the difference, and the difference can be debilitating.

In the 1930s, Barnett Sure at the University of Arkansas conducted hundreds of experiments on the links between nutrition and fertility, for it is in their reproduction that animals manifest nutritional imbalances and deficiencies most dramatically and rapidly. Sure's laboratory animals repeatedly showed that supplementation with synthetic B-complex vitamins interfered with normal reproduction, causing lactation problems, sterility, stillbirths, and infant mortality. The more synthetic vitamins his animals had ingested, the worse their reproductive health.

Synthetic and natural vitamins interact differently with minerals in the body. *Health Alert* editor Bruce West, D.C., warns his patients and readers that the long-term use of synthetic vitamin C (ascorbic acid) depletes copper and tyrosinase levels, which weakens the adrenal glands; high doses of synthetic bioflavonoids may interfere with thyroid function; high-dose synthetic or fractionalized vitamin E can induce gamma or other tocopherol deficiencies and interfere with selenium absorption; and large doses of synthetic or isolated beta carotene can induce powerful carotene imbalances. Dr. West blames the lack of vitamin B_4 in synthetic supplements for many heart problems. This little-known portion of the vitamin B complex was found to have a specific action on the heart and heart muscle. Found in liver, yeast, raw wheat germ, and in supplements derived from these foods, vitamin B_4 is an essential nutrient for circulatory health, and a deficiency can cause arrhythmias and other heart problems.

Unlike its synthetic counterpart, the vitamin C in citrus fruits, acerola cherries, amla berries, rose hips, red and green peppers, and other fruits and vegetables does not disrupt the body's mineral balance. More importantly, ascorbic acid is only one of many chemicals in the natural vitamin C complex; it is not really vitamin C at all. Some vitamin C supplements labeled "natural and organic" are synthesized from corn sugar (glucose), which is not the same as a natural vitamin C complex from whole food. Read labels carefully, and if the source isn't obvious, call the manufacturer and ask how the product is made.

Sometimes referred to as vitamin P, bioflavonoids such as rutin, quercetin, and hesperidin occur naturally in the pulp and peel of citrus fruits, peppers, buckwheat, black currants, algae, and other plants. Because bioflavonoids enhance the absorption of vitamin C, they are often combined in supplements, but the bioflavonoids in a vitamin C product are as likely to be synthetic as the vitamin C itself.

Antioxidant supplements are a big business, and in addition to the well-known combination of selenium and vitamins A, C, and E, antioxidants such as beta carotene, lycopene, lutein, coenzyme Q10, alpha lipoic acid, and proanthocyanidins are sold separately. Any product containing a single nutrient is produced in a laboratory, not from whole foods. When beta carotene failed to protect heavy smokers from heart attacks, headlines condemned vitamin therapies without mentioning that the supplement tested was synthetic, not derived from food.

Critics of isolated nutrients note that taking beta carotene by itself no matter what its source is unnatural, for foods that are rich in beta carotene contain other nutrients that work synergistically to protect health. For example, spirulina contains alpha carotene, beta carotene, zeaxanthin, cryptoxanthin, and other carotenes. Among their other benefits, mixed carotenes have been shown to protect the skin against the harmful effects of ultraviolet radiation and reduce DNA damage, a leading cause of cancer. Carrots, another rich source of carotenes, contain alpha carotene, beta carotene, epsilon carotene, gamma carotene, lycopene, and dozens of compounds that have yet to be identified. As David G. Williams, M.D., explains in his *Alternatives* newsletter, "It would be a serious mistake to think that a single beta carotene supplement would provide the same protection as the combination of carotenes found in carrots."

In response to the increasing demand for natural or food-based vitamins, more manufacturers are supplying them. However, labels are not always easy to decipher. If a label uses the abbreviation USP for United States Pharmacopoeia, this assurance of purity is also an indication that the nutrient was manufactured in a laboratory, not derived from whole foods. Sustained-release or timed-release products are always synthetic, and any label showing that the supplement provides a substantial vitamin dose almost always indicates a synthetic product. If a label advertises nutrients "such as are found in whole foods," it claims to be similar to whole-food nutrients, but it doesn't contain those foods. Supplements that contain whole foods list those foods on their labels.

Americans have become so accustomed to megadose vitamin therapies that the labels of Standard Process supplements, which are derived from whole foods, look like misprints. Cataplex E-2 tablets contain only 2 International Units (IUs) of vitamin E, and the recommended human maintenance dose is two tablets per day. By megavitamin standards, that's nothing. The Wysong product Food-C contains 150 milligrams of vitamin C per capsule, and Nature's Plus brand of chewable Acerola-C Complex contains 250 milligrams of vitamin C per water, while synthetic supplements of the same size contain six to eight times those amounts. How can such small doses have any effect on human health?

The answer lies in how our bodies recognize and deal with nutrients in food (which are familiar and easily assimilated) in contrast to our very different response to synthetic or fractionated supplements. Made from glandular materials and high-selenium yeast, Cataplex E-2 is the most popular Standard Process product, best known for its ability to improve cardiac function, prevent heart arrhythmia and angina, increase the distribution of oxygen through the respiratory system, increase stamina, and help prevent infection. In addition, it prevents common reproductive problems, maintains heart health, promotes efficient detoxification, improves endurance, and helps prevent altitude sickness among mountain climbers.

Wysong's Food-C contains sprouted barley, acerola juice, black currants, grape juice, whole rice syrup, rose hips, composted kelp, orange juice, and green cereal grasses. Instead of a single vitamin, Food-C contains over 115 nutrients including vitamins, minerals, enzymes, bioflavonoids, antioxidants, and essential fatty acids. Nature's Plus Acerola-C Complex contains acerola extract powder, lemon bioflavonoid complex, rose hip extract, black currant concentrate, green pepper extract, and rutin from natural sources, making it another easily assimilated source of related nutrients.

Many excellent supplements make no claims of specific potency. The Vitamin Shoppe's Green Phyters tablets contain organically grown, freeze-dried spirulina, chlorella, barley juice, wheat grass, and alfalfa leaf. Wysong's Salad capsules contain extracts and concentrates of broccoli, brussels sprouts, cauliflower, red and green cabbage, kale, and broccoli sprouts. Neither product claims to contain any measured amount of any nutrient, but both are superior to synthetic supplements of guaranteed potency.

Whole-food supplements are so different from synthetics that label comparisons can be meaningless. More is not necessarily better, and while large doses of synthetic vitamins have been used with success in the treatment of malnutrition, synthetically produced megavitamins are not only unnecessary for perfect health, they can cause nutritional imbalances and adverse side effects.

Another reason to take vitamin supplements derived from whole-food sources is that vitamins work best with other vitamins and minerals, not in isolation. Nutrients in whole foods are more likely to be in balance, as well as compatible with one another, than synthetic, isolated, or fractionated nutrients. The nutritional literature is full of warnings about vitamins and minerals that interfere with each other's assimilation and performance, but these warnings apply to supplements produced in laboratories, not supplements made from whole foods and the thousands of complex chemicals they contain.

MINERALS

Since the late 1800s, America's farm soils have been stripped of their minerals and trace elements. The result is such a severe mineral depletion that the mineral levels of our industrially grown staple crops are insufficient to provide and maintain good health. The most widely used chemical fertilizers contain only two or three minerals, not the seventy-two or more trace elements found in nature.

Mineral deficiencies interfere with vitamin absorption, digestion, and the health of every body system, from the brain's electrical circuitry to the healthy operation of the heart, circulatory system, reproductive organs, skeleton, skin, lungs, and everything else.

Boron is used by the body in trace amounts for calcium uptake and strong, healthy bones. Calcium is essential for bones and teeth, a regular heartbeat, the transmission of nerve impulses, and healthy muscle growth and movement. Chromium is necessary for the synthesis of cholesterol, fats, and proteins and for maintaining stable blood sugar levels. Copper participates in the formation of bones and red blood cells, wound healing, energy production, pigmentation, and healthy nerves. Germanium improves cellular oxygenation. Iodine feeds the thyroid, metabolizes excess fat, and maintains healthy mental and physical development. Iron is the blood's most important mineral, for it produces hemoglobin and oxygenates red blood cells. Magnesium is essential for enzyme activity, and it improves calcium and potassium uptake. Manganese helps metabolize fats and proteins, and it maintains healthy nerves, blood sugar levels, and the immune system. Molybdenum enables the body to utilize nitrogen, and it promotes normal cell function. Phosphorus is essential for bone and tooth formation, heart muscle contraction, kidney function, and cell growth. Potassium maintains stable blood pressure, a healthy nervous system, and a regular heartbeat. Selenium protects the immune system, helps maintain heart health, and improves pancreatic function. Silicon or silica is essential for healthy bones, connective tissue, nails, skin, and hair. Sodium maintains fluid balance and blood pH levels; it is needed for healthy stomach, nerve, and muscle function. Sulfur protects cells, disinfects the blood, resists bacteria, and improves digestion. Vanadium helps maintain healthy cell growth, the formation of bones and teeth, and reproduction. Zinc is needed for protein synthesis, collagen formation, wound healing, prostate gland function, growth of the reproductive organs, and the ability to smell and taste.

Seaweeds such as kelp and dulse provide dozens of minerals, including iodine. Brazil nuts are rich in selenium. Blackstrap molasses and wheat germ contain substantial amounts of magnesium. Fruits, nuts, and vegetables are rich in boron. Kelp, nuts, and seeds are sources of chromium. Avocados and fish are rich in copper. Deep-sea fish contain iodine. Organ meats provide substantial amounts of iron and potassium. Unrefined sea salt contains trace amounts of all nature's minerals.

The advantage to food-derived minerals is that they are easy to assimilate in proportions that living bodies utilize well. Whenever it's necessary to provide a mineral supplement, consider using a liquid or powder that contains most or all of the elements found in nature rather than a product that contains only one, two, or five minerals. Mineral supplements derived from animal sources, plant material, ocean water, or salt lakes are easily absorbed, well tolerated, and in natural balance.

Some of these sources have been called dangerous because they contain small quantities of aluminum, arsenic, cadmium, lead, mercury, and other toxic elements. Although the microscopic amounts in unrefined sea salt have never been shown to affect human or animal health adversely, some manufacturers of concentrated colloidal minerals remove potentially toxic minerals and trace elements from their products.

The claim that plant-derived minerals do not accumulate in the body is supported by research on kelp, some species of which are known for their high arsenic content. Elemental arsenic accumulates in the body, and it doesn't take much to kill someone, but plant-derived arsenic behaves differently. In Japan, which has the world's highest per capita consumption of kelp, tests on human volunteers showed that 100 percent of the arsenic ingested in seaweed was excreted in the urine within sixty hours. In addition to correcting mineral deficiencies, kelp and other seaweeds contain alginates that soothe and cleanse the digestive tract while preventing the absorption of toxic metals such as mercury, cadmium, cesium, plutonium, strontium, and other radioactive isotopes.

AMINO ACIDS

Amino acids are the building blocks of proteins needed to construct every cell of every organ, bone, and fluid in the body. Eight are called essential amino acids because they cannot be synthesized by the body and must be supplied in food or supplements, and the remaining fourteen, called nonessential acids, are formed within the body by essential amino acids. For optimum health, essential amino acids must be provided in the proper balance.

One excellent whole-food source of amino acids is the supplement Seacure (see Resources). Made from deep-sea fish that are predigested by a fermentation process developed in Uruguay, Seacure powder is rich in amino acids and peptides, easily assimilated, and hypoallergenic. In addition to protein, it contains unsaturated fats and mineral ash, including calcium and phosphorus. Seacure is recommended for a variety of conditions in people of all ages to speed wound healing, boost immunity, improve digestion, and relieve joint pain. Its most dramatic effects were shown in extensive tests on premature, underweight, malnourished human infants who were given 1 to 2 grams daily.

Their weight, digestion, and immune functions improved significantly, and in many, allergies disappeared.

KELP AND OTHER SEAWEEDS

Best known for their abundant minerals and trace elements, kelp and other sea vegetables have a nourishing and tonic effect on all the body's systems.

In addition to correcting mineral deficiencies, they contain alginates that soothe and cleanse the digestive tract, improve glandular function, promote rapid hair growth, and correct pigmentation. They are important for healthy reproduction and protect against heart and kidney disease. For information on seaweed's safety, see pages 103 to 104.

Most health food stores offer a variety of North American and Japanese seaweeds, such as nori, also known as laver; kelp, also called kombu; wakame, hijiki, and arame (which are brown); and red dulse, which contains the highest iron concentration of any food source. Agar-agar, known as kanten in Japan, is used as a jelling or thickening agent. For those with digestive problems, sea vegetables are best when cooked for long periods, as in soup stock.

ALOE VERA

The same succulent that offers relief from sunburn, insect bites, and skin irritation is a food supplement. Its juice or gel, which is sold as a beverage, has been shown to improve the skin and hair, increase joint mobility, relieve arthritis symptoms, improve digestion and help clear kidney, bladder, and urinary tract infections.

Quality is an important consideration for aloe vera shoppers, and labels can be difficult to decipher. Juices and gels labeled "cold processed" are actually pasteurized, and most juices and gels contain chemical preservatives. Some are "whole leaf" preparations, which include the laxative outer rind, some contain only the inner gel, and some contain flavoring agents, artificial colors, sugar, high-fructose corn syrup, ascorbic acid (synthetic vitamin C), or other questionable ingredients. The most expensive aloe vera products are powders containing isolated fractions of the plant; the most expensive juices and gels are sold by multi-level marketers, and dramatic advertising claims are common. Look for reputable manufacturers, organically grown aloe vera, and products free of artificial colors, stabilizers, and flavoring agents.

BEE POLLEN, ROYAL JELLY, AND BEE PROPOLIS

Bee pollen is a rich source of amino acids and vitamin B_{12}, and it is widely reported to improve endurance, promote longevity, aid recovery from chronic illness, and help prevent disease. But bee pollen often contains impurities, such as the pollen of ragweed and other allergenic plants. Although bee pollen has been used to prevent allergies (see page 210), it has also been blamed for serious allergic reactions.

Flower pollen, which is collected by hand, does not contain the weed pollens commonly found in bee pollen, thus the risk of allergic reaction is reduced. Flower pollen has been shown to be an effective treatment for prostate enlargement in men, and it is a popular supplement among athletes for improved performance and stamina.

Royal jelly is the substance nurse bees manufacture from pollen to feed the queen bee, who grows substantially larger and lives far longer than her sisters. This concentrated source of nutrients has been marketed as an immune system booster, anti-aging compound, and virility drug. Pure royal jelly is one of the most expensive supplements on the market. Most royal jelly products combine royal jelly with raw honey.

Propolis is sometimes called "bee glue" because bees collect the sap of polar buds and the resin of coniferous trees, mix it with enzymes, beeswax, and pollen, and use it to repair cracks in the hive, coat larval cells, form protective openings that allow only bees to enter the hive, and embalm any rodent that might invade the hive and be stung to death. As a result, despite its warmth and humidity, the interior of a bee hive is more sterile than most hospitals.

Bee propolis is considered one of the strongest natural antibiotics and disinfectants known; it has antibacterial, antifungal, antimicrobial, antiseptic, and antiviral properties. Propolis is widely used to support the immune system and as a specific for cancer, urinary tract infections, throat swelling, open wounds, sinus congestion, bronchitis, gastritis, circulatory disorders, and virus infections such as colds and flu.

Some physicians believe that propolis has a stimulating effect on the thymus gland, which is the master gland of the endocrine system and an immune system regulator. Research conducted in Eastern Europe and Austria indicates that propolis may repair cellular damage caused by X rays, kill cancer cells while leaving healthy cells intact, and rapidly heal stomach ulcers.

WHEAT GRASS, RYE GRASS, AND OTHER CEREAL GRASSES

Cereal grasses are nutritional powerhouses, rich in chlorophyll, amino acids, minerals (especially potassium, calcium, and magnesium), vitamins, enzymes, and protein. They have a strong cleansing action and are popular supplements for detoxification, the correction of nutritional deficiencies, the treatment of cancer, atopic dermatitis, pancreatitis, digestive problems, skin conditions, insomnia, anemia, and respiratory diseases. All cereal grasses have a deodorizing effect, which helps to improve the breath and body odor.

Wheat, rye, oats, kamut, spelt, barley, and other grasses are easy to grow. Books by Ann Wigmore and other raw–diet authorities give detailed instructions. Barley grass is especially recommended because of its high B-vitamin content, but all grasses offer health benefits. Buckwheat lettuce, with its red stems, makes a colorful addition to salads and is a rich source of the bioflavonoid rutin.

Cereal grass products, especially powders, are popular supplements. Powders are convenient, so if you aren't able to grow your own grasses, look for products that are dried at low temperature and grown organically. Wheat grass and barley grass from the Pines company are grown under conditions that produce unusually high concentrations of vitamins and minerals.

Now that an Australian manufacturer has patented an extract of rye grass called Oralmat and tested it against asthma and other illnesses, rye grass may begin to rival wheat grass as an herbal cure-all. Preliminary reports claim that very small quantities (3 drops under the tongue two or three times per day for adults and children) improve not only asthma but allergies, colds, flu, diabetes, and infections caused by viruses, fungi, and bacteria.

Placebo-controlled clinical trials are underway in Australia, with researchers reporting "extremely promising" preliminary results in the treatment of asthma.

Green juices are powerful medicines that should be used sparingly. Too much too fast can cause dizziness, vomiting, diarrhea, and other symptoms of rapid detoxification. To prevent this problem, start with a small amount and let your body adjust before increasing the amount you use.

MICROALGAE

Billions of years ago, algae covered the oceans. The first photosynthesizing organisms on our planet, they are believed to have made the earth hospitable to future life by converting carbon dioxide to oxygen, thus creating our atmosphere. Spirulina, chlorella, and blue-green algae are among the world's most widespread herbs, and in recent years they have become among the most popular. Nearly every brand of supplement has at least two or three products containing microalgae.

Not every strain of algae is edible, but the species sold as food supplements are nontoxic and rich in chlorophyll, amino acids, vitamins, minerals, and protein.

Spirulina, named for its cell's spiral shape, is the only microalgae visible to the naked eye. Spirulina has become popular with vegetarians, athletes, expectant mothers, senior citizens, and others who want to improve or maintain their health. First studied by scientists in the 1940s, spirulina was found to contain 65 to 70 percent protein, the eight essential amino acids, abundant vitamin B_{12}, and other nutrients.

Chlorella, another single-celled algae, derives its name from its high chlorophyll content. Chlorophyll repairs cells, increases hemoglobin in the blood, and speeds cell growth. In addition to being sold by itself, chlorella appears in many products that combine "green" ingredients, such as the other microalgae, wheat or barley grass juice, alfalfa, and green vegetables. Processing that breaks chlorella's cell wall is said to improve assimilation.

Blue-green algae, the popular name for a strain of *Aphanizaomenon*, grows on lakes and ponds. Like spirulina and chlorella, blue-green algae contains chlorophyll, vitamins, minerals, protein, amino acids, and other nutrients.

Are there significant differences between spirulina, chlorella, and blue-green algae? Or between wild harvested and cultivated strains? According to researchers not affiliated with manufacturers, there is little to be gained from comparing their individual merits. Nearly all descriptions of one type's superiority or another's inferiority come from manufacturers' promotional literature. Research conducted in Japan, Mexico, the United States, and other countries indicates that similar results can be expected from all three.

WILLARD WATER

Willard Water, also called catalyst-altered water, is a concentrate sold in some health food stores and by mail (see Resources). John Willard, Ph.D., a professor of chemistry, developed this substance while working in oil fields, and after much experimentation, he patented two forms of the concentrate. Willard Water is sold as a clear or dark concentrate for mixing with "good" water, good being defined as uncontaminated spring water, distilled water, or filtered tap water. The treated water, which reduces stress and improves digestion and the assimilation of nutrients in humans and animals, was the subject of a *60 Minutes* television program in 1980 as well as two subsequent books.

I was interested in Willard Water's ability to destroy chlorine and to act as a preservative and disinfectant, so in 1991, the year he died, I corresponded with Dr. Willard. In a letter dated April 16, he wrote, "In answer to your question, I will give you some information that is not public knowledge. Take ⅓ ounce (10 c. c.) of clear Willard Water extract in 1 gallon of good water (use distilled or deionized water if you're not sure). Put the dilute solution in a mist sprayer and spray it on hair, wounds, food, raw meat, etc., to disinfect. It reacts with the air to become a powerful oxidizing agent and preservative. I have cleaned up two hospitals with very hazardous contamination. In answer to your question regarding its use with raw milk or fresh juice, add one ounce of either clear or dark Willard Water per gallon, or 1½ teaspoons per quart. We discovered this with an old Swiss cheesemaker. Milk tastes richer and keeps fresh longer."

It is easy to add a pinch of unrefined sea salt and a splash of Willard Water concentrate to drinking water and to fresh, raw juice. Willard Water has been used and tested on animals for decades, and the result is a long list of documented improvements with no adverse side effects. The most frequently reported claims from farmers, veterinarians, breeders, trainers, handlers, and pet owners are improved digestion, calmness, improved coat luster and eye sparkle, improved gait, resistance to stress–related illness, and increased immunity. Similar benefits, especially improved digestion, increased mobility, and relief from arthritis, are reported by Willard Water's human users.

COLOSTRUM AND LACTOFERRIN

Colostrum is the first milk a mammal produces after giving birth. This liquid is so rich in immune system support that it protects newborns from infections and intestinal disorders. Colostrum affects thirty-two growth factors including muscle, cartilage, connective tissue, body weight, and lean muscle. Derived from cow's milk, colostrum supplements are reported to enhance immune function. Lactoferrin, one of the immune factors in colostrum, is also sold as an immune-enhancing supplement.

Colostrum and lactoferrin protect the mucous membranes, interfere with the reproduction of harmful bacteria, activate T-cells which attack invading organisms, repair damaged muscle and cartilage tissue, and improve muscle tone. They are recommended for anyone who is ill, susceptible to illness, or recovering from any disease.

GLANDULAR THERAPY

The endocrine system consists of the pituitary, thyroid, parathyroid, and adrenal glands, ovaries, testes, and parts of the pancreas, all of which produce hormones, which are substances that modify the structure or function of other organs or tissue. Unlike sebaceous and sweat glands, which discharge their secretions through tubes or ducts to small local areas, the endocrine glands, which are also called ductless glands, send their hormones directly to the bloodstream, through which they affect tissue throughout the body. For example, the adrenal cortex produces corticosteroids, the pituitary produces growth hormones, the testes produce androgens, and the ovaries produce estrogens and progesterone.

Physicians routinely prescribe synthetic hormones for the treatment of all types of endocrine disorders. Less familiar, at least in the United States, is the use of over-the-counter supplements made from whole, raw glands and organs.

In ancient Greece, Rome, and China, the organs of animals were believed to restore vigor and potency to middle-aged and older people. The first recipient of modern glandular therapy was a woman who in 1931 received injections of an extract made from the parathyroid glands of calves to relieve muscle spasms that resulted from the accidental removal of her thyroid gland and a portion of her parathyroid during goiter surgery. Loss or damage of the parathyroid gland results in a precipitous drop of serum calcium levels which can lead to uncontrollable shaking and death. Within a day of her injection, the patient's serum calcium levels returned to normal, and they remained so with the help of the injections for another thirty-five years.

Radioactive isotope tracing has shown that glandular tissue is absorbed by corresponding glands in the body. For example, if someone ingests raw cellular material from a cow's liver, it will be carried to that individual's liver. In Europe, where physicians have used raw glandular therapy for nearly a century, raw liver supplements are routinely used to treat hepatitis, jaundice, toxemia, cirrhosis caused by alcoholism, and other liver function problems.

Raw kidney supplements treat kidney damage caused by cadmium toxicity, high blood pressure, kidney infections, and kidney stones. Extracts of raw thyroid help stabilize an over- or underactive thyroid, and adrenal gland extracts help repair damage or depletion of the adrenal glands.

In 1983, obstetrician/gynecologist Carson Burgstiner, M.D., contracted hepatitis B from a finger puncture while performing surgery on an infected patient. His acute infection progressed to a chronic illness that lasted for seven years. Frustrated by his inability to heal despite the best of conventional care, and forced by his status as the carrier of a blood-borne virus to restrict his medical practice to nonsurgical procedures, Dr. Burgstiner searched on his own for a cure.

He considered the thymus the key to his problem, for it is widely known as the "master gland" of the immune system. Dr. Burgstiner reasoned that when this crucial gland malfunctions, supplementing the diet with thymus extract might enhance immunity, so he purchased thymic extract and a vitamin-mineral complex at a local health food store. After six weeks of this simple therapy, his blood test for the hepatitis virus was negative for the first time in seven years of repeated testing. The Centers for Disease Control in Atlanta, Massachusetts General Hospital in Boston, and the Scripps Institute in California all confirmed his test results and announced a "spontaneous remission." His surgical privileges were restored.

Dr. Burgstiner, who died before his theory could be proven, devoted the balance of his career to thymus gland research. In patients taking his formula, he documented cures of eighty-four hepatitis B, thirty-four hepatitis C, twenty-eight rheumatoid arthritis, ten multiple sclerosis, and twelve psoriasis cases, as well as the remission of twelve cases of systemic lupus. Thymus gland support is an important factor in treating any illness that involves the immune system.

One of the most familiar glands is the thyroid, for thyroid imbalances are widespread. Hypothyroid (low or deficient thyroid) symptoms include cold hands and feet, low body temperature, fatigue, a slow pulse, fluid retention, slow mental reflexes, and hair loss. Thyroid deficiencies contribute to chronic infections, immune suppression, slow-healing wounds, muscle cramps (especially at night), chronic low back pain, joint aches, anemia, chronic bruising, minor bleeding, excessive menstruation, ulcers, premature aging, life-threatening infections, allergies, depression, and an increased risk of heart disease and the degenerative diseases of old age.

Conversely, a good supply of thyroid hormones in the blood helps people feel younger, better, more energetic, and more intelligent, while preventing many illnesses and disorders.

A simple way to test for hypothyroidism was developed by pioneer thyroid researcher Broda O. Barnes, M.D., Ph.D. To prepare for the test, shake down an oral thermometer and leave it where you can reach it as soon as you wake up in the morning. Immediately on awakening, place the thermometer in your armpit and lie with your arm close to your body for ten minutes, then check your temperature. After five consecutive mornings, average your waking underarm temperature. If the average is lower than 97.4 degrees Fahrenheit (some say 97.6 degrees Fahrenheit), you probably have an underactive thyroid even if blood tests show normal thyroid function. Other physicians recommend using an oral thermometer under the tongue every three to four hours during the day for a week or two. An average daily temperature that is consistently below 98.6 degrees Fahrenheit indicates an underactive thyroid.

Patients taking synthetic thyroid hormones require careful monitoring. Natural thyroid, which has fewer side effects, is available by prescription, but many respond well to whole-thyroid supplements which do not contain hormones. The nutrients in glandular extracts support and help balance glandular action. Thytrophin from Standard Process, and Thyroplex, a supplement designed by Jonathan Wright, M.D. (see Resources), help prevent hypothyroidism.

Hyperthyroidism, the opposite condition, is the result of an overactive thyroid gland. In conventional medicine, the diagnosis of hyperthyroidism is based on blood tests, and the standard treatment (irradiation, surgery, and/or prescription drugs) has such significant and permanent side effects that many question its wisdom, especially because a fast metabolic rate is not necessarily unhealthy. In some populations, such as Alaskan Inuits and Mexico's Yucatan Indians, the average metabolic rate is 25 percent faster than what American physicians consider normal. Excessive thyroxine (thyroid hormone) in one person may be the correct amount in another.

The same whole-thyroid supplements that help repair an underactive thyroid help lower an overactive thyroid. In addition, the daily consumption of fresh, raw cabbage juice and other cabbage-family vegetables, including collard greens, brussels sprouts, broccoli, and cauliflower, depress thyroid function. These foods, which are best avoided or eaten in small amounts by someone with an underactive thyroid, are recommended for those with a rapid resting pulse (over 120 beats per minute), bulging eyes, and other symptoms of hyperthyroidism.

Glandular therapy may sound unusual, but glands and organs have been part of the human diet for millennia. Only recently have American tastes turned away from liver, kidneys, tripe (stomach), sweetbreads (pancreas and thymus), heart, and other organs that supply the same endocrine tissue as today's glandular supplements. Many chronic conditions that cause discomfort can be corrected with their help. For recommended glandular products, see the Resources. For tonic herbs that help balance hormone levels and support the body's glands and organs, see page 151.

CHAPTER FIVE

Medicinal Herbs

By far, the world's most widely used natural therapy is herbal medicine. Every culture on every continent has experimented with local plants and developed a tradition of diagnosis and use based on experience and observation.

My teacher, Rosemary Gladstar, offers sensible advice to those who are new to these old traditions. "In order for herbs to be effective," she says, "they must be used with consistency. This is probably the most difficult aspect of herbalism for people in the twentieth century. In our age of quick fixes and instant medicine, the old art of brewing and using herbal tea seems antiquated and time-consuming." On the contrary, she explains, it's really easy and practical. So is the use of herbal powders, capsules, tinctures, extracts, salves, essential oils, and other products.

"The real advantage of medicinal herbs," explains Gladstar, "is that they work both gently and thoroughly. Herbs don't have the side effects of pharmaceutical drugs, but they are powerful medicines nonetheless."

Herbalist Deb Soule agrees. "The information the public receives about herbal medicine is often trendy and superficial," she says. "Because our culture is so accustomed to the methods of allopathic medicine, it is easy to look at herbs as simple replacements for pharmaceutical drugs, but this is a mistake. Herbs don't suppress symptoms the way drugs do; they go deeper, to the source of a health problem, and they are usually gentler and slower acting. When you use whole-plant ingredients like blossoms, leaves, and roots, you're using versatile materials that don't have to be measured like prescription drugs."

ON THE SAFETY OF HERBS

To say that herbs are controversial is to make an understatement. Cautions about their potential toxicity abound, and the U.S. Food and Drug Administration (FDA) is quick to issue warnings. Is the user really in danger?

In a few cases, yes, but poisoning is far more likely to be caused by the accidental ingestion of a toxic plant than the intentional use of a medicinal herb. For example, many people become seriously ill or die every year as a result of eating incorrectly identified mushrooms. Occasionally someone dies after eating a toxic plant that was mistaken for a medicinal plant, as happened to one couple who misidentified foxglove as comfrey. Foxglove, the source of digitalis, is highly toxic. A few years ago, an herbal product manufactured in the United States was recalled after users became ill from a European foxglove that was misidentified as plantain. Some herbal products imported from China and Taiwan are contaminated with pharmaceutical drugs and other questionable ingredients. Responsible herbalists guard against accidental or intentional adulteration by growing or collecting the herbs they use, buying from reputable sources, and testing herbs purchased in bulk for their quality, purity, and identification.

At the same time, an herb can be 100-percent natural, correctly identified, organically grown, and correctly processed, yet still pose a hazard.

Ethnobotanist David Winston borrows a description from Native American medicine to introduce the wide range of properties herbs possess. "In the Cherokee tradition there are three types of herbs," he explains. "There are food herbs, which can be used in large quantities and which are very unlikely to create any type of adverse reaction. There are medicines that require more knowledge and which should be used for specific conditions for a specified period of time because they are stronger and have the potential to cause adverse reactions if used incorrectly. Then there are poisons, which can cause serious adverse reactions up to and including death. This last group of herbs should be used only by people trained in their safe use and administered in very small doses."

Category 1: Safe "Food" Herbs

Dandelion, stinging nettle, chamomile, burdock root, calendula, lavender, echinacea, ginseng, raspberry leaf, parsley, garlic, cilantro, oregano, dill, sage, and rosemary are examples of food herbs that have a long history of safe, effective use. Many herbs with a more medicinal reputation belong to this category, too, such as hawthorn berry, which is usually classified as a heart medicine; saw palmetto berry, which prevents prostate enlargement; and valerian root, a relaxing nervine. It includes herbs described as tonics, which gradually restore and strengthen the entire system; alteratives, which gradually cleanse the blood; and adaptogens, which gradually restore balance throughout the body; all of which work best when taken daily for months or years. Most of the herbs mentioned in this book belong to Category 1.

Category 2: Powerful Medicines

As more serious medicines, cascara sagrada and senna leaf are examples of the second category. These laxative herbs should be used in small doses and for a limited time to avoid bowel irritation, diarrhea, dehydration, and mineral imbalances. Other examples are the stimulant herb Ma huang (ephedra), which opens the bronchial passages but should not be used by people with high blood pressure, and herbs that contain caffeine, such as green tea, guarana, and kola nut. Large doses of the catalyst herb lobelia, which is both a nerve tonic and respiratory aid, can cause vomiting, and large doses of the relaxing herb kava kava can interfere with coordination.

Category 3: Toxic Herbs

Herbs from this category, such as the previously mentioned foxglove, are true poisons. These herbs can be powerful medicines in minuscule doses but are not appropriate for home use. Aconite, deadly nightshade, hemlock, jimsonweed, mayapple, skunk cabbage, and pokeweed are other examples. You will never find Category 3 herbs in popular tea blends.

Category 4: Topical Irritants

Some common herbs cause skin irritation and must be handled with care. For example, raw garlic applied to the skin to treat fungal infections has caused burns and skin damage sufficiently serious to send people to hospital emergency rooms. Powdered mustard and cayenne pepper are rubefacient herbs, which increase blood circulation to the skin when applied as a traditional plaster to alleviate respiratory congestion or in a cream to relieve joint pain, but both can cause redness, a burning sensation, and irritation. Cayenne is especially irritating to the eyes, so keep hands away from the eyes after handling hot peppers. Water will not remove cayenne's irritating oils, but vegetable oil will. Apply any cooking oil to relieve discomfort.

Essential oils are so concentrated that they require careful handling. Clove bud, cinnamon bark, cassia, oregano, thyme, and savory essential oils are significantly irritating to the skin and can cause burning, blistering, and discomfort. Other essential oils can cause redness and irritation when treated skin is exposed to sunlight.

Before applying fresh herbs or essential oils to the skin, review instructions and recipes to be sure they are prepared and applied correctly. If you have sensitive skin, apply a small amount of any unfamiliar herbal preparation or diluted essential oil to the inside of the knee or elbow as a patch test to check for allergic reactions. The patch test is recommended for children, the elderly, and anyone with a history of dermatitis, hives, or skin sensitivities. Inspect the area every fifteen minutes for an hour, then every few hours for twenty-four hours. If the preparation causes blistering, burning, pain, or an allergic reaction, use a different herb or essential oil, or dilute the preparation further and try again.

HERBS AND PREGNANCY

Most herb books contain a list of herbs to avoid during pregnancy. While some of these lists are exceedingly cautious, it makes sense to avoid therapeutic doses of medicinal herbs during pregnancy, childbirth, and nursing, except for those specifically recommended or so nontoxic that they don't pose a threat. Angelica, black cohosh, blue cohosh, motherwort, and yarrow are known to stimulate uterine contractions. Fennel, a popular digestive herb, is often listed as an herb to avoid during pregnancy because of its estrogen-like activity. Wormwood in small amounts is unlikely to cause harm, but large quantities of powdered wormwood are certainly not recommended during pregnancy.

Many herbs that are safe in their natural state are far more likely to cause problems when concentrated as essential oils. During pregnancy, it's best to use the safest and most gentle essential oils and to obtain them from distributors who specialize in therapeutic-quality organically grown or wildcrafted essential oils (see Resources). These oils are more expensive than the essential oils sold in health food stores and cosmetic counters. Because they are so concentrated and potent, they can be used sparingly, which makes them more affordable. A single drop has therapeutic benefits, and essential oils can be diluted in a carrier oil, vegetable glycerine, or alcohol for external application or bath use. An experienced aromatherapist can answer your questions about the safe, effective use of essential oils during pregnancy.

Many books warn that aloe vera should not be used during the first trimester of pregnancy. However, this caution is based on the effects of evaporated and processed *Aloe ferox* (Cape aloe from South Africa) and *Aloe vulgaris* (the common aloe of North Africa and Southern Europe), which are concentrated laxatives with abortifacient properties. The juice or gel of aloe vera, an entirely different plant, does not cause uterine contractions and does not interfere with pregnancy, childbirth, or nursing.

Sometimes scientific research adds to the confusion sur-rounding herbs and their effect on reproduction. In March 1999, researchers at the Loma Linda University School of Med-icine in Loma Linda, California, made headlines when they re-ported that four best-selling herbs might cause pregnancy risks. Hamster eggs and human sperm exposed to dilute solutions of St. John's wort, *Echinacea purpurea*, and *Ginkgo biloba* suffered damage, including a reduced ability of sperm to penetrate an egg, changes to the genetic material in sperm, poor sperm via-bility, and, in the case of St. John's wort, mutation of a tumor suppressor gene. Of the herbs tested, only saw palmetto, which is commonly taken by men to relieve the symptoms of an en-larged prostate, did not damage eggs or sperm in the doses tested, although it did reduce the viability of sperm exposed to the herbal preparation for seven days.

The researchers noted that there is no evidence suggesting that people taking the recommended dosages of these herbs are adversely affected, for no data exist on the concentrations of these herbs in semen or blood serum, and the herbal doses tested do not represent amounts that actually reach eggs or sperm in people taking them. Many mainstream scientists have criticized the study's design as well as the media's misrepresentation of its results. One wonders what the researchers would have discov-ered if they had tested the effects of city tap water, cola bever-ages, aspirin, chemical preservatives, and artificial flavors on eggs and sperm.

Practicing herbalists and midwives who have studied medic-inal herbs are your best sources of information regarding the safe use of herbs and essential oils during pregnancy.

THE PROBLEM WITH
"DANGEROUS PLANT" LISTS

As a result of the explosion of interest in natural remedies, America's newspapers, magazines, and television news programs have interviewed experts of every description regarding the effectiveness, use, and safety of herbs. Because medicinal herbs are unfamiliar to most physicians, pharmacists, health care professionals, and scientists in the United States, these authorities often repeat inaccurate or incomplete information. In some cases, an herb is labeled dangerous because its berries are poisonous, because of a single documented allergic reaction, or because laboratory animals that had ingested large amounts suffered adverse side effects.

It is always disconcerting to see Category 3 plants like aconite, deadly nightshade, foxglove, hemlock, jimsonweed, mayapple, and pokeweed listed as though health food stores sell their dried leaves for tea brewing, but some physicians who truly don't know the difference warn their patients away from all medicinal herbs because a few are dangerous. Others, with nothing but previously published warning lists to guide them, pass on information that was never accurate or which has been disproved since the list was compiled. Some misrepresented herbs are especially helpful in treating conditions that cause pain and discomfort, and some widely used herbs can cause allergic reactions. Here are examples.

Aloe Vera

Although the wide use of this popular herb has made health-conscious Americans aware of its benefits, it is sometimes listed as unsafe for internal consumption because the bitter juice of its inner rind has a laxative effect. Most bottled aloe vera juice or gel contains little or none of this ingredient. To use home-grown aloe vera or leaves purchased from a market or health food store (Hispanic markets often sell large aloe leaves), carefully pare the rind and rinse away any yellow or orange sap before adding the gel to fruit or vegatable juice in your blender. If one brand of aloe vera juice or gel has an undesired laxative effect, try another. Dried, whole-leaf aloe vera in capsules is more likely to have this effect because whole-leaf preparations contain the laxative sap, and dried powders are more concentrated than the juice or gel. Aloe vera is a Category 1 herb.

Arnica (*Arnica montana*)

An important first-aid item, arnica tincture (an alcohol extract) is best known for its dramatic effect on bruises—and for its "external use only" labels. Dian Dincin Buchman, Ph.D., is one of many American herbalists who caution against using arnica internally. In her popular book *Herbal Medicine*, she writes, "I must warn you that arnica is never to be used on open flesh wounds externally. Arnica may only be used on unbroken skin!"

European physicians have long prescribed arnica tea or tincture as a cardiac agent, but it is such a powerful heart stimulant that it can be dangerous. As a result of its history and frequently published warnings, most American herbalists know that arnica should be used only externally and only on unbroken skin.

But by taking such a cautious approach, say some experts, users deprive themselves of arnica's most important potential, for in small doses, arnica can stop internal bleeding and stimulate healing, especially after trauma injuries. For emergency use, take 10 drops arnica tincture two to four times daily, diluted in water. For children, use 2 to 5 drops twice per day.

According to Ed Smith, a highly regarded herbalist and researcher and founder of Herb Pharm, an herbal products manufacturer, arnica is a specific for internal injuries and the complications they cause. Smith finds no justification for the warnings on arnica products, and in addition to its internal use, he recommends applying it to bleeding wounds and other injuries to reduce swelling, pain, and bruising.

Arnica is a Category 2 herb which should be used carefully. But, its potential benefits far outweigh its risks. Be sure the tincture is made with grain alcohol, not isopropyl (rubbing alcohol) or denatured alcohol. If in doubt, check with the manufacturer.

Burdock Root (*Arctium lappa*)

This common Japanese vegetable is found in sushi bars, health food stores, Japanese markets, and many herbal formulas. Reports of its toxicity stem from a single instance in which a batch of burdock was contaminated with belladonna root, which contains three toxic alkaloids, including atropine. The incident was never repeated, but some medical authorities continue to list burdock as toxic. Burdock is a Category 1 herb.

Castor Oil

The ornate castor plant, a popular garden accent, can cause allergic reactions, and its elaborately patterned seeds are so poisonous that a single one can kill a dog or small child, but the castor oil that is sold for pharmaceutical purposes does not contain the seed's toxins. Taken internally, castor oil is a purgative laxative, which can be useful in an emergency, but it is seldom recommended for internal use. Instead, this plant is valuable for its external application in castor oil packs, described on page 176.

Chamomile (*Matricaria chamomilla, Anthemis noblis*)

Chamomile is often blamed for allergic reactions, especially in people who have ragweed allergies. In the past hundred years, only five cases of chamomile allergy have been reported in the medical literature, and some research suggests that chamomile actually helps alleviate allergic reactions such as hay fever. Chamomile is an exceptionally safe Category 1 herb with important digestive, anti-inflammatory, and relaxing benefits.

Chaparral (*Larrea tridentata*)

Chaparral received unfavorable publicity in the late 1980s when it was blamed by the FDA for acute toxic hepatitis, and a voluntary ban on the herb's sale was initiated by sellers. In the years that followed, no additional cases of chaparral toxicity could be found. After an extensive review of chaparral's history by medical experts with specialties in gastroenterology and hepatitis, followed by discussions with FDA officials, the Board of Trustees of the American Herbal Products Association voted in 1995 to rescind its recommendation that members suspend the sale of chaparral. The herb is once again widely available.

Chaparral tea repels and helps eliminate worms and other

parasites. It can be applied to wounds and itching skin to speed healing; it kills most viruses, including the herpes virus, and it has potent cancer-fighting properties. Despite its safety and effectiveness, chaparral continues to appear on "dangerous herb" lists. While most herbalists suggest using herbs other than chaparral for patients with liver disease, it is an excellent Category 1 herb. Some chaparral extracts have been treated to remove the plant's controversial oxidative components (see Resources), but teas and tinctures containing untreated chaparral are safe for long-term use.

Coltsfoot (*Tussilago farfara*)

In 1987, a Swiss infant born with a severely damaged liver died. Every day of her pregnancy, the mother drank an expectorant tea containing coltsfoot. The tea contained senecionine, a pyrrolizidine alkaloid, but its source was uncertain; it may not have been coltsfoot. As a precaution, the German government placed a one-year moratorium on the sale of coltsfoot. No other cases of potential coltsfoot toxicity were discovered and the ban was repealed. Coltsfoot preparations, including tinctures, teas, and syrups, are effective in treating respiratory illnesses, including coughs, bronchitis, and other lung conditions. Despite its proven safety, coltsfoot is often listed as a dangerous herb that causes liver damage. It is, instead, a Category 1 herb.

Comfrey (*Symphytum officinale*)

Comfrey has been removed from most health food store shelves and tea blends because it contains pyrrolizide alkaloids (PAs) that, when isolated and consumed in large doses, can cause liver damage and cancer in rats. In hundreds of years of use, no cases of human problems with comfrey were ever documented, but in 1984, a woman who had been taking comfrey-pepsin tablets developed liver toxicity and, since then, three additional cases of human liver disease have been reported in people who took the herb.

Because of the plant's long history of safe use, some herbalists continue to use it in the treatment of gastritis, diverticulitis, irritable bowel syndrome, spastic colon, peptic ulcers, duodenal ulcers, leaky gut syndrome, and Crohn's disease. Others, alarmed by laboratory tests, recommend that comfrey be removed from all herbal preparations. "These are the extremes of the comfrey controversy," says Rosemary Gladstar, "but most herbalists take a middle ground, recommending small amounts for internal purposes and large amounts externally. As for me, until the evidence and 'hard facts' are much more compelling, I will continue to use comfrey judiciously for myself and my clients. The Austrian company that conducted the original tests that alarmed everyone has verified that the tests were inconclusive, and in Japan, where comfrey's alkaloids were first discovered, doctors continue to recommend comfrey for cirrhosis of the liver. I believe that the small amounts of pyrrolizide alkaloids found in comfrey are balanced by this herb's abundance of the cell proliferant allantoin and by calcium salts and mucilage, all of which are nutritious to the cells and serve to counteract the cell-inhibiting actions of the pyrrolizide alkaloids."

PA-free comfrey tinctures are available for those who wish to take advantage of the plant's exceptional properties without the risks (if indeed there are any) posed by pyrrolizide alkaloids. See the Resources.

For those who grow comfrey or buy unprocessed comfrey leaf or root tea, small quantities are unlikely to cause problems. When taking larger quantities of untreated comfrey to speed the healing of broken bones or treat digestive disorders, add milk thistle seed, an herb whose flavonoids help prevent the liver's absorption of PAs. For external use, comfrey is a Category 1 herb. The only warning to keep in mind is that it is not recommended for use on deep puncture wounds because the rapid skin healing it causes may trap infection beneath the surface. For internal use, it is prudent to consider comfrey a Category 2 herb.

Echinacea (*Echinacea purpurea, E. angustifolia*)

A powerful immune system stimulant, echinacea has been shown to increase phagocytic (white blood cell and macrophage) activity even after the user stops taking it. Although many herbalists prefer to use echinacea in large doses at the beginning of an active illness, early American and modern German research has shown it to be safe and effective for long-term oral consumption.

Is echinacea dangerous? Rumors have circulated in Europe since a 1996 German television program claimed that allergic reactions to echinacea caused three deaths. A prominent German scientist investigated these cases and proved that echinacea was not a factor. Over ten million units of echinacea products are sold annually in Germany, where no allergic reactions have been documented. Between 1993 and 1996, the U.S. FDA received eight reports of adverse effects in people who took echinacea, including hepatitis, abdominal distress, and arsenic poisoning. In some cases, the products contained other substances or were adulterated, and the FDA was unable to verify a connection between echinacea and any of the eight reported problems.

Recent speculation that echinacea interferes with conception or poses a risk to unborn children is based on test-tube experiments described on page 123 and is not supported by clinical experience in humans, pets, or laboratory animals. Reports of its long-term use interfering with immune function are based on the incomplete translation of a German clinical study in which an accompanying graph showed a marked increase of phagocytic activity of human granulocytes for the first five days of treatent followed by a gradual drop over the next five days, without noting that the echinacea was given for only five days, not ten. Echinacea, which is Europe's most widely prescribed botanical medicine, is exceptionally safe and effective.

Ginseng (*Panax ginseng*)

The most famous herb of all, ginseng is controversial partly because in 1979 the *Journal of the American Medical Association* published an informal poll of 133 psychiatric patients who were also ginseng users, who consumed up to 15 grams of ginseng daily (over twice the highest recommended dose), inhaled or injected the herb (bizarre applications by any standards), or took it with large amounts of coffee. Some of them took a different plant altogether. Most of these users experienced symptoms ranging from morning diarrhea to nervousness, insomnia, and elevated blood pressure. All of these side effects are associated with caffeine, and the unrelated plant "desert ginseng," which several took by mistake, is a laxative. This extremely misleading report continues to be quoted in medical journals as evidence of ginseng's adverse side effects. Ginseng is a Category 1 herb.

Kava (*Piper methysticum*)

This South Pacific herb, also known as kava kava, has quickly become one of America's fastest-selling supplements. Kava reduces stress and anxiety, helps focus attention, promotes restful sleep, and relaxes muscles. However, large doses have adverse side effects, including a temporary lack of coordination and, over time, an unattractive skin rash. In Utah and California, police have arrested drivers whose coordination was impaired after drinking ten to sixteen cups of kava tea. Kava is not recommended for those who are clinically depressed. It is a very safe Category 2 herb for short-term use in small amounts.

Licorice (*Glycyrrhiza glabra, G. uralensis*)

Familiar to Americans as a black candy with an anise flavor, licorice is native to the Mediterranean and parts of Asia. Its root has been used since antiquity as a sweetener and to treat coughs and respiratory problems, but licorice is best known today as a cure for ulcers.

Unfortunately, a compound called glycyrrhizin in licorice causes water retention (edema) in an estimated 20 percent of those who take large doses. Deglycyrrhizinated licorice extracts were developed so that ulcer patients could take the herb without this side effect.

Deglycyrrhizinated licorice (DGL) is used to treat peptic and duodenal ulcers as well as canker sores. Most American drug stores sell DGL products as digestive aids. Whole-root licorice with its glycyrrhizin intact is still used by herbalists to treat adrenal weakness and coughs.

Licorice is a Category 2 herb. Because long-term use of untreated licorice root can cause sodium and water retention, hypertension, potassium loss, dizziness, headaches, and impaired kidney function, it should not be used by those with hypertension, kidney disease, or edema. This includes imported licorice candy that contains natural licorice extract. (Most American licorice candy is artificially flavored and does not contain licorice extract.) Untreated licorice root products should not be combined with stimulant laxatives or diuretics that contribute to potassium loss. Deglycyrrhizinated licorice (DGL) is a Category 1 product. It has no known adverse side effects.

Lobelia (*Lobelia inflata*)

Also known as Indian tobacco, lobelia has a long and colorful history. It is an important ingredient in respiratory blends because it causes the immediate relaxation and expansion of contracted bronchial tubes as well as the esophagus, glottis, and larynx. It is also a relaxing nervine or tonic for the nerves. When blended with other herbs, lobelia acts as a catalyst, increasing their effectiveness.

However, lobelia's nineteenth-century promoters became so popular that the medical establishment of the day brought charges against them. As several authorities on the history of herbal medicine have shown, witnesses fabricated testimony blaming lobelia for a host of problems that it doesn't cause. The herb's tarnished reputation survives today, with reference books and FDA reports claiming that it is poisonous, toxic, dangerous, and potentially fatal. These accusations, which stem from nineteenth-century trials conducted in the United States and England, remain unproven.

According to Mark Blumenthal, executive director of the American Botanical Council and publisher of the journal *HerbalGram*, some scientists want to ban lobelia because in large doses it causes vomiting, even though, as he notes, "it has nowhere near the toxic potential of aspirin or ibuprofen." Lobelia is a very safe Category 2 herb.

Ma Huang or Chinese Ephedra (*Ephedra sinica*)

Widely used in the treatment of respiratory disorders and often combined with caffeine for use in weight loss supplements, Ma huang contains the alkaloids ephedrine, pseudoephedrine, and norpseudoephedrine. All are strong central nervous system stimulants that are more powerful than caffeine but less potent than amphetamine. Taken in excessively large doses, ephedrine produces heart palpitations and, in some people, a feeling of euphoria.

This last side effect made ephedra a recreational drug. To produce a "legal high," manufacturers of Herbal Ecstasy and similar products combined large quantities of Ma huang with other herbs, especially those that contain caffeine. The result was a form of "speed" that can be fatal. Between 1993 and 1996, about four hundred people reported adverse reactions to ephedra-based products, ranging from dizziness to strokes, and at least fifteen died. Ma huang-related deaths among college students spurred a movement to ban the herb's sale, and public health officials weighed the dangers of recreational overdoses against the benefits of products containing small amounts of Ma huang.

Although several states outlawed the sale of Ma huang as a recreational drug, in 2000 the FDA withdrew its proposed restrictions of Ma huang products. In responsibly formulated herbal blends taken as directed, Ma huang has an impressive record of safety and effectiveness. It is not recommended for those with high blood pressure, heart disease, or anxiety, and it should not be combined with large quantities of caffeine. Ma huang is a Category 2 herb.

Pennyroyal (*Mentha pulegium*)

A member of the mint family, pennyroyal has long been used as a digestive aid. Warnings about its safety stem from the death of an infant who was given daily doses of pennyroyal leaf tea and from the misuse of its highly concentrated essential oil. Full-strength pennyroyal leaf tea should not be given to infants or small children, but tea blends containing pennyroyal are safe for older children and adults.

Because of its reputation as an abortifacient, some women have attempted to end their pregnancies by taking pennyroyal essential oil internally. This is a dangerous undertaking, because pennyroyal oil is toxic to the liver, and some women have died as a result. Essential oils are so concentrated that only a few are recommended for internal use, and pennyroyal isn't one of them. Pennyroyal is a Category 2 herb; pennyroyal essential oil is a Category 3 herb.

Peppermint (*Mentha piperita*)

Peppermint tea and peppermint essential oil have been used for centuries to help relieve indigestion. Because it is very concentrated, peppermint essential oil in large amounts can cause gastrointestinal distress and burning, and neither peppermint tea nor its essential oil is recommended for heartburn because it relaxes the muscles that allow acid to move from the stomach to the esophagus. Peppermint is not recommended for infants because its menthol may cause a choking reaction. For older children and adults, peppermint is a Category 1 herb.

Psyllium Powder

This popular bulking fiber, the key ingredient in Metamucil and similar products, has caused skin and respiratory allergies in psyllium manufacturing plants and in hospitals or nursing homes where attendants stir it into juice for hundreds of patients at a time. To avoid frequent and prolonged exposure to psyllium, avoid spilling the powder, and wear a pollen mask or keep the head averted while measuring and stirring. When taken with insufficient liquids or in large quantities, psyllium can cause or contribute to intestinal blockages. Psyllium is a Category 2 herb that should be used with common sense.

Sassafras (*Sassafras albidum*)

A traditional ingredient in spring tonics and a flavorful digestive aid, sassafras contains safrole, a substance that the FDA blamed for causing cancer in laboratory rats in the 1950s. Safrole is also found in nutmeg, black pepper, and mace, but these seasonings were never implicated. Because safrole is not soluble in water, someone drinking sassafras tea can ingest very little of it, and no case of liver damage from sassafras tea has ever been reported. The southeastern United States, where most sassafras tea is consumed, has a lower liver cancer rate than other parts of the country. Sassafras is a very safe Category 2 herb.

Wormwood (*Artemisia absinthium*)

Wormwood, a member of the artemisia family, has a long history of safe use in people and animals as a digestive aid and treatment for parasites. Because wormwood essential oil is a key ingredient in the infamous liqueur absinthe, which was outlawed in many countries a hundred years ago, some authorities consider wormwood dangerous in any form, warning that it causes convulsions, loss of consciousness, and hallucinations. Fresh or dried wormwood in the amounts usually recommended does none of these things. Even wormwood essential oil, which is highly concentrated, is considered by the FDA to be safe for internal use when sold as a flavoring agent from which the psychoactive principles have been removed. Wormwood is a Category 2 herb.

Yucca (*Yucca species*)

A member of the lily family, yucca has several common names, including soapweed. You can literally wash your clothes with it. The same saponins that give yucca its soapy properties help relieve the inflammation of arthritis, but they also irritate the stomach lining and intestinal mucosa. The digestive distress that results from too much yucca can cause pain or bloating, and prolonged exposure to saponins can cause anemia as well as disturbances of the central nervous system. Other foods that contain saponins include soybeans, alfalfa, oats, legumes, potatoes, garlic, and beets.

Yucca is a Category 2 herb. It is safe in small doses but should not be taken in large amounts, more often than four or five times per week, for more than a month or two at a time, or during pregnancy. It is a good idea to avoid other saponin-rich foods when using yucca.

HOW TOXICITY IS REPORTED

Most warnings about toxic herbs stem not from experience but from theory and the ways in which herbs are researched, regulated, and reported. Herbs contain hundreds of chemicals, and it is not unusual for an herb with a long history of safe, effective use to contain one or more chemicals that, when isolated and fed in large amounts to laboratory animals, cause serious problems.

Toxicologists determine the relative safety of a drug by weighing its benefits against anticipated risks. Aspirin and ibuprofen cause between ten thousand and twenty thousand human deaths per year, a statistic that receives little publicity and which is regarded by most health care professionals as unfortunate but acceptable in light of the pain relief these drugs provide. In contrast, herbs used medicinally are so rarely toxic that a single adverse side effect makes headlines.

Some confusion in the United States stems from the FDA's "GRAS" or "Generally Recognized as Safe" list, which contains about two hundred herbs commonly used as extracts, flavorings, oils, and seasonings. An additional two hundred herbs in common use do not appear on the list, such as slippery elm bark, burdock root, arrowroot, catnip, coltsfoot, echinacea, flaxseed, goldenseal root, gotu kola, hibiscus flowers, horsetail, uva ursi, stinging nettle, saw palmetto berry, skullcap, senna, tormentilla, blue vervain, and yellow dock root. Such herbs are not unsafe; they are simply unlisted.

The Herb Research Foundation is one of the organizations gathering scientific data pertaining to herb safety from around the world. If you have questions about the safety of any herb or if you'd like information about an herb's uses, contact the HRF (see Resources).

Common sense and education are your best guides to herb use. Don't use an herb without learning about it first. The safest herbs may be those you grow yourself using organic methods, plants you harvest from areas that are free of pesticides and far from the automobile exhaust of busy highways, and dried herbs purchased from reputable sources, labeled organically grown or wildcrafted. Unfortunately, most herbs imported into the United States are fumigated on arrival, a consideration for anyone using herbs medicinally. No discussion of herb safety would be complete without a mention of this concern.

INTERACTIONS

Can one herb interfere with the effects of another? Is it dangerous to mix herbs? What about pharmaceutical drugs? Can herbs interfere or create complications when taken with other medications?

Adverse side effects caused by Category 1 and 2 herbs are

extremely rare, either alone or in combination. Some physicians combine orthodox therapies with herbs and essential oils with good results, often reducing or eliminating prescription drugs in the process. For the treatment of serious conditions, medical supervision is always recommended.

Herbs that reduce blood sugar levels may change a diabetic patient's need for insulin. Castor oil so dramatically increases the skin's absorption that any drug, herb, or chemical applied at the same time will quickly move into the bloodstream. Herbs that thin the blood, such as garlic and ginkgo, may change a patient's response to anticoagulant drugs. These herbs should be used with caution by patients with blood-clotting disorders and, to avoid surgical complications, they should be discontinued before elective surgery. Both garlic and ginkgo speed postoperative healing, and they are safe to resume after surgery. In addition, herbs that contain saponins, such as garlic and yucca, should not be used together in large quantities because of potential damage to red blood cells or digestive disturbances.

The PDR for Herbal Medicines, an annual Physicians' Desk Reference first published in 1998, devotes several pages to possible drug/herb interactions, only a few of which involve herbs from Categories 1 and 2. Feverfew (*Tanacetum parthenium*), which is recommended for arthritis and migraine headaches, increases the antithrombotic effects of aspirin and warfarin sodium; white willow (*Salix* species), a natural form of aspirin, should be used with caution with nonsteroidal anti-inflammatory drugs and salicylates; psyllium husk powder, flaxseed, and laxative herbs can interfere with the absorption of other drugs taken simultaneously; brewer's yeast (*Saccharomyces cerevisiae*) in combination with MAO inhibitors may increase blood pressure; medication that increases uric acid levels may decrease the effects of uva ursi (*Arctostaphylos uva-ursi*), an herb used to treat urinary tract infections; and the long-term use of rhubarb root (*Rheum palmatum*) in combination with cardiac glycosides may increase their effect due to potassium loss.

Other books describe possible herb/drug interactions in more detail, but problems involving the most widely used herbs, especially when they are taken as teas or other whole-plant preparations, are extremely rare. As practicing herbalists are fond of noting, the most widely used over-the-counter and prescription drugs are far more dangerous than almost any combination of medicinal herbs.

Now that pharmaceutical companies advertise to the public, popular magazines provide interesting juxtapositions. Typically an article warning readers not to take medicinal herbs because they are dangerous is sandwiched between ads for prescription drugs that list hundreds of adverse side effects, including many that are incapacitating or fatal.

STANDARDIZED PRODUCTS

Few topics have so polarized American herbalists as the controversy surrounding standardized products. Standardized extracts, which are the herbal preparations most similar to pharmaceutical drugs, are guaranteed to contain a specific, isolated amount of an herb's key ingredient. For example, many standardized echinacea extracts contain a minimum of 4 percent echinacosides, which are thought to stimulate immune function. Typical ginkgo extracts contain 24 percent ginkgoflavonglucosides, which are believed to enhance memory, and many St. John's wort extracts are standardized to contain 0.3 percent hypericin, which is believed to be its mood-elevating ingredient.

Despite their official looking labels, standardized extracts are not more effective or more "scientific" than crude, whole-plant extracts. Plants are complex, not simple, and medicinal herbs contain thousands of chemicals. Because they are so complicated, scientists don't know how they work. For example, according to scientific literature, the active ingredient in valerian has changed five times in the last decade. Most extracts of St. John's wort (*Hypericum perforatum*) are standardized for hypericin, but new research suggests that an entirely different constituent, hyperforin, may be responsible for the herb's effectiveness as an antidepressant. As a result, some St. John's wort supplements are now standardized for hyperforin instead of hypericin. It is possible that neither hypericin nor hyperforin accounts for the herb's effectiveness in conditions that are not mood-related. St. John's wort can repair nerve damage, as evidenced when the fresh herb or an oil infusion of its blossoms is applied to a nerve-damaging injury and the person makes a rapid, full recovery, and the herb repairs damage to the skin caused by burns or other injuries. St. John's wort was traditionally used as a blood purifier, mild diuretic, uterine tonic, and regulator of menstrual cycles, functions that are likely to involve still other active ingredients.

Standardized extracts were created because of the need for consistent experimental doses in scientific studies. Because their similarity to chemically manufactured drugs has impressed conventional physicians, standardized extracts are often promoted as superior, safer, and more effective than competing products. They may not be so. Herb books always mention that the consumption of large quantities of St. John's wort, which is an invasive weed in the Pacific Northwest, has caused photosensitivity (an allergic reaction to sunlight) in cattle. These books usually warn that St. John's wort might cause a similar reaction in humans while noting that no such cases have been documented. During the last few years, however, some clinical herbalists have reported seeing photosensitivity in patients taking standardized St. John's wort extracts, a side effect that disappeared after the patients replaced their standardized products with crude whole-plant tinctures. These reports remain anecdotal, but they suggest that some standardized products may cause more adverse side effects than their crude, whole-plant equivalents.

According to James Green, director of the California School of Herbal Studies, this development is not surprising. "When you pull one ingredient out and throw the rest away," he says, "you lose the plant's synergy. If you use the whole plant, which has a variety of nutritional components, you experience a gentle process that produces a wide variety of beneficial effects and the side effects are minimal, if any at all. Isolate a single ingredient and you experience all kinds of adverse side effects because the body isn't able to recognize or deal with isolated ingredients."

Green's main objection to standardization is that it places the emphasis on science. "When we embrace standardization because it's scientific," he explains, "we accept the notion that science will make things better, and in doing so we disempower ourselves. Herbalism thrives in the home. People should realize that the plants are out there, they're whole and perfect the way they are, and you can go out and identify a plant, harvest it, and make your own medicine for yourself and for your family. You have all the personal power you need to make the finest medicines available, and your result can be a medicine that's superior to anything technology can offer."

HOW TO JUDGE AN HERB'S QUALITY

The best dried herbs are fragrant, flavorful, colorful, and pungent. They don't look like shredded hay or smell like cardboard. They are dried at a low temperature with lively air circulation and stored away from heat, light, and humidity, the enemies of all dried herbs. The best herbs for medicinal use are grown organically or wildcrafted from pollution-free sources, then handled with care at every step of their drying and storage. By their look, smell, and taste you can recognize these plants—the peppermint is obviously peppermint and the chamomile is obviously chamomile.

Here are some simple rules to keep in mind as you evaluate dried herbs. The larger the piece, the longer it lasts. Herbs begin to lose their flavor as soon as they are ground into powder. The more a leaf is exposed to heat, light, the open air, and humidity, the faster it loses its healing properties as well as its taste.

This information will help you answer a commonly asked question: "How long can a dried herb be kept before it loses its effectiveness?" The answer is, "It depends." While many herbs should be replaced after a year, the most sensible rule is to look, smell, touch, and taste. Roots and bark hold their fragrance, color, and taste longer than delicate leaves and flowers, yet even blossoms and leaves can retain their herbal identity for much longer periods if properly stored.

INTERNAL AND EXTERNAL APPLICATION

Herbs have many uses. They can be added fresh or dried to food, brewed as teas, swallowed in capsules, or concentrated in liquid extracts called tinctures. Plant material can be applied topically as a poultice; teas can be applied as cold compresses or hot fomentations. Herbs can be added to oils to create oil infusions for topical application. Salves are thickened oil infusions.

Herbal Teas

Although capsules and tinctures are convenient, teas provide an herb's medicinal benefits in a form that's easy to assimilate even when digestion is impaired.

The simplest teas are infusions, also known as tisanes (pronounced tee-SAHN). An infusion or tisane is made from fresh or dried herbs and hot water. Chamomile, peppermint, and most other leaves and blossoms lend themselves to this method. For best results, use distilled, filtered, or bottled spring water, not chlorinated tap water. The water should be heated to just below the boiling point.

Proportions of herbs to water for most beverage teas are:

1 teaspoon dried herb per cup of water
1 to 2 tablespoons fresh herb per cup of water
4 to 6 teaspoons dried herb per quart of water
¼ to ½ cup fresh herb per quart of water

These are guidelines, not hard and fast rules. For example, use less of an herb that is dense and heavy, more of an herb that is light and fluffy, less of an herb that is fragrant and in excellent condition, and more of an herb that is old and tired. Everything depends on the quality of the herb and the tea's purpose.

A decoction is a simmered or boiled tea. Roots and seeds are brewed by this method, though some roots with volatile oils require the more gentle infusion procedure, and some leaves must be simmered instead of steeped. Always check individual descriptions in herbal reference books.

To brew a decoction, bring plant material and cold water to a boil in a covered pan, then lower the heat and simmer gently for ten to fifteen minutes. Remove the pan from the burner and let the tea stand another five to ten minutes before straining and serving.

Alternatively, place cold water and herbs in a glass canning jar, seal it tightly, and place it in a water-filled pan that is large enough to accommodate the jar and a small rack. The rack is used to elevate the jar enough to keep it from rattling and breaking when the water boils. Cover the pan, bring the water to a boil, reduce heat, and simmer gently for at least one hour. This method can be used to brew any type of tea, infusion, or decoction, for it maintains a steady temperature, protects fragile plant constituents, and prevents evaporation. Traditional Chinese ginseng cookers, which are ceramic jars with small feet, work the same way.

A medicinal tea is a concentrated tea for therapeutic purposes made by increasing the proportion of herbs to water, increasing the brewing time, or both. Use up to twice as much plant material as for a beverage tea; the quantity depends on the quality of the herb, so if the herbs are potent, you may need less. Let the tea stand until cool or let it stand overnight before straining. Store leftover tea in the refrigerator for no more than two or three days. For medicinal purposes, the tea should be strong and fresh.

Another way to brew a medicinal tea is to make an attenuated infusion, a method used by New York herbalist Billie Potts. "For attenuated infusions," she says, "I steep the herb in boiling water, let it stand for three to four hours, and then, without removing the plant material, gently reheat the tea at a slow simmer for one hour."

For most conditions, the recommended dosage is 1 to 3 cups beverage-strength herbal tea per day for adults and up to 1 cup for children. Medicinal-strength teas are used as needed, the quantity depending on the condition.

Tinctures

Tinctures are liquid extracts that concentrate and preserve an herb's medicinal and nutritional properties. These are the preparations you see in the small, amber glass bottles with eyedropper tops that line health food store and herb shop shelves. Because they are simple to use, easy to store, portable, and effective in small quantities, tinctures are very popular.

They are also expensive. Even though doses are usually measured in drops, it doesn't take long to go through a 1-ounce bottle. You can save substantial sums of money by making your own from fresh, whole herbs when they are available.

To tincture fresh herbs, loosely pack a glass jar with plant material and cover it with vodka, vegetable glycerine, or apple cider vinegar. To tincture dry herbs, fill the jar only one-third full to leave room for expansion, add a slightly larger amount of liquid, and every few days add more as needed to keep a 1-inch margin of liquid above the herbs. Leave the jar in a warm place for four to six weeks, shaking it every few days. The longer a tincture stands, the more concentrated it becomes.

Strain the liquid and store it in cobalt blue or amber glass jars in a cool, dark location. Dispense in eyedropper bottles. To make a double-strength tincture, strain the liquid into a glass jar containing additional fresh or dried plant material, and repeat the process.

For most conditions, the recommended tincture dosage for adults is 15 to 30 drops (¼ to ½ teaspoon, or 1 to 2 dropperfuls) three times daily. For children, use about 2 drops per 10 pounds of body weight three times daily. Smaller amounts produce good results if the tincture is double-strength and made from superior-quality fresh herbs. Additional tincture may be needed if the product is weak or made from inferior-quality herbs.

Herbal Capsules

Because they are easy to administer in food or capsules, crushed dried herbs and herbal powders are popular supplements. If you need a special blend of herbs in capsules, some of the mail-order herb companies listed in the Resources blend and encapsulate custom orders for a nominal fee. Try to buy herbal capsules from retailers whose stock rotates quickly or who powder herbs for capsules as needed. Powdered herbs lose their potency when exposed to heat, light, or humidity.

The most concentrated capsules are made from supercritical extracts. Supercritical extraction uses compressed carbon dioxide gas to dissolve the oily fractions of herbs that are oily in nature, like feverfew, ginger, kava kava, oregano, rosemary, saw palmetto berry, and St. John's wort. It takes 250 pounds of fresh ginger to produce one pound of supercritical extract, which is free of solvents. Some plant chemicals, such as the hyperforin resins in St. John's wort, are unstable in alcohol but have a long, stable shelf life in supercritical extracts.

Oil Infusions

To make an oil infusion, such as an oil for treating ear infections or in preparation for salve-making, you can use the stove, an oven, the sun, or an electric cooker. Although any carrier oil can be used, olive oil is the standard medicinal infusion oil.

Fresh chopped garlic and fresh or dried mullein blossoms are traditional ingredients in ear oils for adults and children. If mullein blossoms are not available, use garlic by itself.

Cover the plant material with olive oil and heat it gently in the top of a double boiler above simmering water, or in a closed glass jar set on a rack in a pan of simmering water for one to two hours or longer. If using dry herbs, additional oil may be needed as the plant matter absorbs it. Use enough oil to cover the herbs completely; start with 2 cups oil to 1 cup dried herbs and adjust the proportions as desired. Fresh herbs, which should be allowed to wilt before use, will absorb less liquid, so simply cover with oil.

Strain the oil through cheesecloth, store it in tightly sealed glass jars, and transfer some to a rubber-tipped eyedropper bottle for easy application. Warm the bottle in hot water before applying several drops to each ear. This herbal ear oil treats mild ear infections, swimmer's ear, and related conditions.

To make a solar infusion, let fresh plant material wilt slightly to reduce its water content, then loosely pack a clean glass jar with fresh herbs (or fill a jar halfway with loosely packed dried herbs), then fill it to the top with oil, clean the top of the jar so that no oil or plant material interferes with a tight seal, put the lid on tightly, and leave the jar in the hot sun for several weeks or months.

My favorite oil for salve-making is a blend of olive oil with fresh St. John's wort blossoms, calendula blossoms, and chopped, wilted comfrey that stays outdoors from July through October. The unusually potent healing properties of this oil, which the St. John's wort colors a deep red, may be due to its prolonged photosynthesis or to the effect of continual sunlight and moonlight.

Another way to infuse herbs in oil is to use the oven. Pour olive oil over fresh or dried herbs in a stainless steel pan, cover with foil, and bake at low heat (200 to 250 degrees Fahrenheit) for two or more hours, or at a higher temperature for a shorter time. Check the pan from time to time to prevent scorching or burning. The oil is "done" when it takes on the color and fragrance of the herbs. Electric turkey roasters, slow cookers (Crock-Pots), and other heat sources also work well.

When ready to use, strain the oil through cheesecloth and add a few drops of tea tree oil or grapefruit seed extract as a disinfecting preservative. Pour into a clean glass jar, label with ingredients and date of preparation, and store away from heat and light. Stored correctly, infused oils last for years, though most herbalists prefer to make them annually for maximum freshness. Note that these oils are for external use only. Discard any oil that becomes rancid.

Herbal Salves

To turn an herbal oil into an herbal salve, just add beeswax. One of the best all-purpose salves you can make begins like the oil on page 151 with fresh or dried comfrey, calendula blossoms, and St. John's wort blossoms. Either infuse oils separately or pour olive oil over the combined plants (equal proportions are nice, but they work well in any combination) and heat until the oil absorbs the color and fragrance of the plants. The more comfrey you use, the darker green the oil will be; the more calendula, the more yellow; and the more St. John's wort blossoms you use, the deeper red.

Basic Salve Recipe

1 cup infused oil (see page 149)
½ teaspoon tea tree oil
¼ teaspoon grapefruit seed extract
    Several drops essential oil (lavender or other)
1 ounce beeswax

Combine ingredients in a double boiler or over very low heat until the beeswax has melted. Test the salve by placing a spoonful in the refrigerator. As soon as it hardens, check to be sure the salve is soft but not runny. If it's too soft, add more beeswax; if too hard, add more oil. Pour into clean baby-food jars or other similar-sized containers. Herbal supply catalogs sell small tins for salve.

This antiseptic, analgesic, soothing salve speeds the healing of cuts, burns, fungal infections, dry or cracked skin, abrasions, and other wounds.

TONIC HERBS

Although many herbs are used to treat specific illnesses or conditions, such as feverfew for migraine headaches, some herbs have such a general restorative effect that they are called tonics.

Tonic herbs strengthen the entire system and restore normal tone and health. Nettle, dandelion, ginger, raspberry leaf, and red clover are examples of herbs that, when taken daily, have a tonic effect on the entire body and help repair its systems directly or indirectly.

The term *adaptogen* describes a tonic herb that strengthens the immune system by strengthening its adaptive response to physical, chemical, and biological stress. Ginseng root (*Panax ginseng*) was the first herb to be described in this way, and now the list includes Siberian ginseng root (*Eleutherococcus senticosus*), foti (*Polygonum multiflorum*), astragalus root (*Astragalus membranaceous*), ashwaganda (*Withania somnifera*), schisandra berry (*Schisandra chinensin*), and holy basil (*Ocimum sanctum*). These herbs have been shown to speed wound healing, decrease fatigue, improve focus and concentration, increase stamina and endurance, repair glands and organs, and accelerate recovery after exercise. Many have anti–inflammatory and digestion–improving properties as well.

The action of adaptogen herbs is often contradictory, with the same herb reported to lower as well as raise blood pressure. This is because an adaptogen herb's action is corrective: it brings the body into balance. If the blood pressure is too high, an adaptogen herb gradually reduces it; if it's too low, the herb gradually raises it. All tonic and adaptogen herbs have a gentle, balancing effect. Their action is much slower than that of prescription drugs, but over time they help correct, reverse, and cure many types of conditions. Tonic and adaptogen herbs work well in a holistic health plan. They are not symptom–specific. They repair the entire body by stimulating healing from within.

CHAPTER SIX

Essential Oils and Aromatherapy

MOST AMERICANS ASSOCIATE aromatherapy with perfume, but the use of essential oils is also a branch of medicine—and it has been for thousands of years. The ancient Greeks, Romans, and Egyptians made use of fragrant oils in baths, massage therapy, and other health treatments.

The volatile oils that give plants their fragrance can be extracted, usually by steam distillation, to concentrate and preserve their substance. The resulting essential oils have profound physical, mental, and emotional influences.

Modern aromatherapy was born in the 1930s, when the French chemist René-Maurice Gattefossé burned his hand in a laboratory experiment and plunged it into the nearest liquid, a vat of lavender essential oil. To his surprise, the pain stopped immediately, and the burn healed quickly without scarring. Gattefossé spent the rest of his career researching essential oils and their effects on mind and body. Other researchers and therapists contributed their findings, and today aromatherapy is a discipline practiced in France by medical doctors and by aromatherapists around the world.

Essential oils are so concentrated that they are measured by the drop. Some essential oil bottles dispense one drop at a time, or you can use your own eyedropper. Eyedroppers with a rubber bulb at one end are recommended for measuring purposes only, not for storage, because essential oils dissolve rubber.

When following a recipe that calls for larger quantities, such as a teaspoon or fraction of a teaspoon, don't rely on tableware because teaspoons vary in size, and don't estimate fractions. Use metal measuring spoons sold for kitchen use, and test them first with drops of water. One teaspoon equals 60 drops. Some aromatherapy texts give formulas in metric units, which require measuring devices calibrated in milliliters. One milliliter equals approximately 12 drops, and 1 teaspoon equals approximately 5 milliliters.

Product quality is an important consideration in therapeutic aromatherapy. While expensive oils are not necessarily superior, inexpensive oils are suspect. Many products labeled "pure essential oil" are of inferior quality, adulterated with synthetic ingredients, or mislabeled. Poor-quality essential oils can cause adverse side effects, or they may simply be ineffective.

For best results, use therapeutic-quality essential oils, such as those sold by companies listed in the Resources at the end of this book. Unlike essential oils produced quickly in large batches under high pressure from commercially grown, pesticide-treated crops which are then standardized by chemical treatment or blending, therapeutic-quality oils are distilled slowly in small batches at atmospheric pressure from organically grown or wildcrafted herbs. They are never standardized, so their qualities vary from batch to batch and from year to year like those of vintage wines.

Some essential oils have such different chemistries that they are labeled according to chemotype. For example, rosemary (*Rosmarinus officinalis*) is available in three chemotypes. Camphor-type rosemary from Spain and Croatia is recommended for muscle pain, cramps, nervous tension, and exhaustion, but it is not recommended for use by children under ten or pregnant women. Cineole-type rosemary from North Africa is a stimulating herb that promotes digestion and is recommended for catarrhal conditions and as a component in blends that are released into the air; when used appropriately, it is safe for children and during pregnancy. Verbenone-type rosemary from Corsica is well tolerated by the skin, has cell-regenerating properties, and is an effective treatment for incipient bronchial infections and colds, but it is inappropriate for children and pregnant women.

Thyme (*Thymus vulgaris*) has four chemotypes. If genuine (it is often distilled from *Thymus zygis* rather than *Thymus vulgaris*), thymol-type thyme is an extremely versatile agent against infection, but because it causes skin irritation, it should not be applied externally. Thujanol-type thyme has stimulating, tonic, and antiviral properties, and it is mild and nonirritating. Linalol-type thyme is both a strong antiseptic and mild on the skin. In *Advanced Aromatherapy: The Science of Essential Oil Therapy,* Kurt Schnaubelt, Ph.D., director of the highly regarded Pacific Institute of Aromatherapy, writes that the gentleness and antimicrobial effects of linalol-type thyme made it an overnight classic. It is a pleasant tonic for nervous exhaustion, "irreplaceable" in skin care, and effective against *Candida albicans* and *Staphylococcus*. Geraniol-type thyme is a luxury oil with strong antiviral effects. It is recommended for use in bronchitis, viral intestinal infections, and insomnia.

In contrast, the rosemary and thyme oils sold in most retail stores have an unknown provenance and chemistry.

SAFETY AND TOXICITY

Some essential oils are so potentially toxic that they are best avoided by the home user. These include the essential oils of rue, santolina, mugwort, thuja, wormwood, hyssop, pennyroyal, sage, and camphor.

Some essential oils make the skin unusually sensitive to sunlight and should not be applied topically. These include bergamot, bitter orange, khella, lemon, lemon verbena, and mandarin. The essential oils of cinnamon, cloves, oregano, and thymol-type thyme are so caustic and irritating to the skin that they can cause burning, even when diluted. The essential oil of peppermint can be applied topically to small areas, such as the forehead or temples, but it should not be used on infants under the age of three because it can irritate respiratory passages.

Dr. Schnaubelt warns that essential oils containing high ketone levels should not be used by pregnant women or children under age ten. These include anise, atlas cedar, basil, eucalyptus, verbenone-type rosemary, sage, spike lavender, and yarrow.

Some of these essential oils can be used in small amounts in blends containing other essential oils and large quantities of carrier oil or other diluting agents. The safe use of potentially toxic essential oils requires therapeutic-quality products and careful study. See the Bibliography and Resources.

DIFFUSING ESSENTIAL OILS

There are many ways to use essential oils, but the most popular and safest is to enjoy their fragrance by releasing them into the air. This can be done with an apparatus called a diffuser (available from aromatherapy companies), or essential oils can be sprayed into the air from a spray bottle, dropped onto a ceramic or paper ring (another aromatherapy supply) that is warmed by a light bulb, or simply dropped onto a cold light bulb that, when turned on, releases the fragrance. Deodorant, antiseptic, and respiration-enhancing oils are commonly used in this manner, although heating an essential oil destroys some of its properties. When sprayed or diffused at cool temperatures, essential oils can disinfect an entire room, eliminating bacteria, viruses, fungi, and molds as well as unpleasant odors. The essential oils of cinnamon, clove, eucalyptus, garlic, lavender, onion, tea tree, and thyme are powerful antiseptics. These and other disinfecting essential oils can be used alone or blended. They can be added to wash water when cleaning kitchen or bathroom floors and surfaces, diluted to make inexpensive but effective air sprays, and added to liquid soap to give it antibacterial properties. See the disinfecting formulas on pages 163 and 164.

When inhaled, the essential oils of nutmeg, lemon, anise, citronella, palmarosa, pine, fennel, thyme, and eucalyptus have an expectorant effect and help treat chronic coughs. Minimal doses produce maximum effects, so best results are obtained when just enough essential oil is used to produce a very faint scent. The concentration of essential oils absorbed during inhalation falls by half within thirty to forty minutes, making this method of application extremely safe even when repeated frequently. Essential oils can be diffused or sprayed into the air, or a drop can be placed on a tissue or paper towel and placed nearby.

The essential oils of lavender, melissa (lemon balm), *Eucalyptus citriodora*, lemon verbena, citronella, and lemon have a calming, sedative effect. These essential oils help relieve insomnia when released into the bedroom or applied in small amounts to sheets or bedclothes.

The essential oils of allspice, angelica, French basil, borneol, cardamom, cinnamon leaf, citronella, coriander, cumin, eucalyptus, ginger, jasmine, peppermint, spearmint, nutmeg, rosemary, sage, vetiver, violet, or ylang ylang can be diffused or sprayed into the air to lift the spirits, maintain energy levels in the afternoon, and prevent fatigue.

Some aromatherapy companies sell blended essential oils in small containers that can be held under the nose to help increase energy, reduce stress, control one's appetite, boost confidence, improve concentration, relieve anxiety, or help one derive other benefits.

TOPICAL APPLICATIONS

During the last fifty years, two very different approaches to therapeutic aromatherapy have evolved. In England, essential oils are seldom applied full-strength and are almost never taken orally. Instead, for most conditions, they are diluted in large amounts of vegetable oil and applied externally. Nearly all aromatherapy books carry detailed instructions for diluting essential oils before applying them to the skin. Most recommend diluting 3 to 5 drops of essential oil in 1 tablespoon vegetable oil, which results in a blend that is between 1 and 2 percent essential oil and 98 to 99 percent carrier oil. This dilution is both extremely safe and economical.

In France, essential oils are sometimes diluted, but they are often applied full-strength, and they are frequently swallowed. To French aromatherapists such as Daniel Penoel, M.D., one of the world's foremost authorities on the therapeutic uses of essential oils, the gentle English approach is suitable when full-strength oils would irritate the skin, but is far too cautious to be effective in the treatment of active infections and serious illnesses.

In *Advanced Aromatherapy,* Dr. Schnaubelt describes a general treatment for infectious illnesses that has three phases. The first three days of treatment emphasize essential oils with mucolytic and expectorant qualities to cleanse the mucous membranes; in phase 2 (days 4 to 7), essential oils with bactericidal and fungicidal components eliminate remaining pathogens; and in phase 3 (days 8 to 21), essential oils with sesquiterpene-alcohol and sesquiterpene-ketone content support convalescence.

In *Natural Home Health Care Using Essential Oils,* Dr. Penoel describes what he calls intensive aromatic therapy, which he recommends for acute infectious diseases such as colds and flu. Blends of carefully selected essential oils (15 to 20 drops at a time) are applied to the soles of the feet, which have been warmed with a hair dryer to facilitate absorption, every twenty minutes for an hour, then every thirty minutes for four hours, and as needed after that. In addition, the patient dilutes the same oils in honey and adds it to herbal tea, places drops of the blend on bed linens and nightwear, and sprays or diffuses the essential oils around the room.

Another way to apply full-strength essential oil to the skin is in the shower. Dr. Schnaubelt recommends applying 12 to 25 drops of undiluted essential oil to warm, wet skin, distributing it over the entire body. "Because of their lipophilic quality," he says, "essential oils will be absorbed instantaneously, and the shower can be continued within fifteen to twenty seconds." This treatment, like Dr. Penoel's intensive aromatic therapy, requires therapeutic-quality essential oils. Potentially toxic essential oils and those that cause skin irritation should be avoided.

A first-aid tip: If tea tree oil or any other essential oil causes eye irritation, or if you accidentally spill a full-strength essential oil on yourself, someone else, or an animal, use any vegetable oil, such as a carrier oil or cooking oil, to dissolve and remove it. Water will not remove an essential oil.

If you spill an essential oil on fabric or furniture, relax. Pure essential oils dissolve quickly without leaving a mark or stain.

DILUTING ESSENTIAL OILS

Carrier oils are vegetable oils used to dilute essential oils. Almond, jojoba, peach kernel, apricot kernel, sesame, and other seed and nut oils are popular examples. For best results, carrier oils should be cold-pressed rather than chemically extracted and from organically grown crops.

Adding an essential oil to a carrier oil is an easy way to create massage oils, skin cleansers, first-aid treatments, and natural beauty products.

In *The Complete Book of Essential Oils and Aromatherapy*, an excellent introduction to the subject, English aromatherapist Valerie Ann Worwood, Ph.D., recommends adding 2 to 5 drops of essential oil to 1 teaspoon carrier oil, which is 6 to 15 drops per tablespoon, or 48 to 120 drops per ½ cup. The result is a blend that is 3 to 8 percent essential oil.

See the 10-percent tea tree oil solution on page 163 for an example of a carrier oil dilution.

Water-Soluble Dilutions

Because essential oils do not dissolve in water, an intermediate step is needed before they can be diluted with herbal tea, aloe vera juice, water, or other nonfat liquids.

When essential oils are first dissolved in alcohol, glycerine, sulfated castor oil, soap, or any other water-soluble solvent, they disperse in water without floating to the top. Small quantities of essential oil can be added to salt with the same result, as in bath salts. Although rubbing alcohol (isopropyl alcohol) will dissolve essential oils, it has its own strong fragrance and is toxic when swallowed. For these reasons, vodka and other grain spirits or brandy are the alcohols of choice in aromatherapy.

For an example formula, see the water-soluble 7-percent tea tree oil solution on page 163.

TEA TREE OIL

Even people who know nothing about aromatherapy have heard of tea tree oil. Thanks to the efforts of Australian importers, the essential oil of *Melaleuca alternifolia* is widely sold, and this versatile product has so many uses that it belongs in every medicine cabinet and first-aid kit.

Full-strength tea tree oil is recommended for topical application, but a patch test is always a good idea when using a product for the first time, especially for those with a history of sensitive skin reactions. Place a drop of undiluted tea tree oil inside the elbow, on the inside of the upper arm, or on the back of the knee. Check it after fifteen minutes, thirty minutes, and at intervals through the next twenty-four hours. If it causes redness, itching, swelling, or irritation, try a different brand (look for a superior-quality tea tree oil labeled eco-harvest, organic, or wildcrafted), or dilute the oil as described on page 163 and try again.

Full-strength or diluted tea tree oil can be applied to skin lesions, insect bites, rashes, burns, abscesses, boils, cuts, abrasions, canker sores, pimples, rashes, infected wounds, and fungal infections. Like eucalyptus oil, which it resembles, tea tree oil is a specific for the respiratory system as well as an all-purpose disinfectant. Australian and British research conducted in the 1930s showed that a 15-percent tea tree oil solution is as effective as the full-strength oil in killing yeast cells, mold, bacteria, and viruses. More recent laboratory tests have shown that concentrations as low as 1 percent are effective against streptococcus and other gram-positive bacteria, *E. coli* and other gram-negative bacteria, and several fungi.

Tea tree oil now appears in soaps, shampoos, hair conditioners, toothpastes, mouthwashes, dental floss, toothpicks, hand lotions, disinfectant wipes, insect repellents, ear drops, foot powders, deodorants, and skin care products. Synthetic tea tree oil is used by some manufacturers, so check labels to be sure you're using *Melaleuca alternifolia* from Australia.

Because pets find its turpentine taste unpleasant, tea tree oil is sometimes recommended for application to body parts that an animal chews or licks incessantly, such as the leg or tail. Holistic health guides often list full-strength tea tree oil as appropriate for use on a pet's insect bites, burns, infected wounds, cuts, ringworm, and other fungal infections. However, temporary paralysis caused by the use of undiluted tea tree oil has been reported to the National Animal Poison Control Center following such use on dogs and cats. Symptoms, which occurred within two to eight hours of application, included depression, weakness, incoordination, and muscle tremors. The reaction disappeared within three to four days.

Even diluted essential oils are too concentrated for use on cats, but they are unlikely to cause problems for dogs or small children if used sparingly. Apply as needed, but keep tea tree oil away from the eyes and mucous membranes, and use full-strength tea tree oil on children and dogs in very small amounts.

10-Percent Tea Tree Oil Solution
(Oil Dilution)

Use this procedure to dilute any essential oil in a carrier oil. Recommended for topical application.

Add 1 tablespoon full-strength tea tree oil to ½ cup (4 fluid ounces) carrier oil. Stir to mix well. Pour into an amber glass bottle and label. Attach a rubber eyedropper to the bottle with a rubber band for convenient application. Do not use a rubber eyedropper cap for storage because essential oils dissolve rubber.

7-Percent Tea Tree Oil Solution
(Water Dilution)

Use this procedure to dilute any essential oil in water, tea, aloe vera gel, or other nonfat liquids. Recommended for disinfecting household surfaces and topical use.

Add 1 tablespoon full-strength tea tree oil to 2 ounces (4 tablespoons) vodka, other grain alcohol, vegetable glycerine, or sulfated castor oil. Shake or stir well and let stand for 10 seconds. If a film of oil floats to the top, add more liquid and shake again. When no oil floats to the surface, pour the solution into a measuring cup and add enough aloe vera juice or gel, herbal tea such as comfrey or calendula, pure water, or any combination of aloe, tea, and water to fill the cup to the 6-ounce or ¾-cup mark. At that point, your solution will be approximately 7 percent tea tree oil.

To make a 15-percent solution, the strength tested in the Australian research of the 1930s, increase the amount of tea tree oil to 2 tablespoons.

Water-soluble solutions of essential oils are the foundation of many aromatherapy products, from soaks and lotions to air sprays. Use the above procedure to dilute any essential oil in a water base. If small amounts of essential oil separate later, simply shake the product before using.

This tea tree oil solution can be sprayed on kitchen and bathroom surfaces, into air ducts or air-conditioning units, and on telephone receivers and mildewed shower walls. It can be added to laundry wash–water or simply sprayed into the air.

Deodorant Air Spray

Recommended for the removal of odors and as an all-purpose air freshener.

Combine 6 parts lavender, 3 parts terebinth, 2 parts lemon, and 1 part mint essential oils.

Use full-strength in a diffuser or dilute with vodka, glycerine, or sulfated castor oil and water for use in a plastic spray bottle; then spray the air, avoiding pets, children, and food.

According to French aromatherapist Nelly Grosjean, this blend, manufactured in France under the brand name Fresh-tonic, satisfies the greatest number of users with its strong, fresh smell and antiseptic action.

A WARNING ABOUT DISINFECTANTS

Manufacturers know that "antibacterial" is a magic word in the United States, which is one of the world's most germ-phobic nations. For years we have used antibacterial soaps, shampoos, sprays, sponges, and mouthwashes. Now we are buying antibacterial toys, paper towels, bedsheets, toothbrushes, high chairs, and other products.

Unfortunately, despite advertising claims to the contrary, growing up in a sterile environment is not a healthy way to live. Public health officials are beginning to warn that the excessive use of antibacterial products is detrimental to adults and even more so to children.

In June 2000, the American Medical Association urged the federal government to regulate the manufacture and sale of the more than seven hundred antibacterial soaps, lotions, and other household products on the market. These disinfectants do not kill all bacteria, only those that are most susceptible, leaving behind whatever bacteria are strong enough to survive and multiply. Surviving bacteria can mutate and develop a resistance to antimicrobial products and antibiotic drugs which may be transferred to dangerous pathogens.

Just as troubling is the damage antibacterial products do to young children. Sterile environments prevent the normal development of a child's immune system, which needs exposure to germs in order to function properly. During their first year of life, babies need exposure to bacteria and other agents of infection in order to produce T-1 helper cells, which make antibodies to dangerous microorganisms. If a baby's environment is too clean, the production of T-1 helper cells is not adequately stimulated and the immune system overproduces T-2 helper cells. These create antibodies to allergens, potentially resulting in lifelong allergies or asthma.

Antibacterial soaps, sprays, and other treatments are best reserved for use when someone in the household is ill or has a compromised immune system, or during times of exposure to colds, flu, or other infectious diseases.

Chemical disinfectants contribute to the development of supergerms because their simple molecular structure makes it easy for microorganisms to adapt and survive. This is why the most widely used disinfectants have been shown to kill only the most susceptible germs, thus disrupting the natural balance of microorganisms. However, essential oils contain so many complex chemicals that bacteria, viruses, fungi, and other microorganisms are unable to adapt to them, especially if they are exposed to more than one. Instead of using tea tree oil by itself, consider alternating tea tree oil with solutions of the essential oils of myrrh, pine, cloves, juniper berries, oregano, and thyme; teas brewed from sage and chaparral; or dilute solutions of liquid grapefruit seed extract. All of these are potent disinfectants.

At the same time, remember the warnings of immunologists, and don't use essential oils or other antibacterial products to prevent your child's exposure to the outside world. The more a developing immune system is challenged by bacteria, viruses, and other microorganisms, the more it is able to protect the person from illnesses of every description, not just in childhood but throughout life.

HYDROSOLS

Steam distillation produces a by-product that is one of the fastest growing segments of the aromatherapy industry. Called a hydrosol, hydrolat, flower water, floral water, herb water, or distillate, this liquid retains the fragrance and other water-soluble components of the leaves, roots, stems, seeds, or blossoms that produced it.

Now appearing in prestigious cosmetic lines as key ingredients in personal care products, hydrosols can be used in place of water in any formula, lotion, creme, shampoo, bath gel, spray mist, foot soak, mask, or scrub. Lavender, rose geranium, lemon balm, and rosemary hydrosols are beginning to replace some chemical ingredients in some commercial products.

Hydrosols are best described as a cross between highly concentrated herbal teas and very dilute essential oils, giving them unique healing properties. In addition to being therapeutic, hydrosols are extremely safe. They can be applied to infants, children, the elderly, and animals such as kittens, birds, puppies, rabbits, and other pets. In addition, unlike most essential oils, they are safe for internal consumption.

Although they do not require refrigeration, hydrosols should be stored away from heat and light. Few retailers carry hydrosols because of their size, storage requirements, and short shelf life. However, as many as fifty therapeutic-quality hydrosols are offered by companies listed in the Resources. True hydrosols, which do not contain preservatives, are fragile. Keeping hydrosols in spray bottles allows them to be used without exposing them to air and bacteria.

"Cleanliness is essential," says Suzanne Catty, who is one of the world's leading authorities on the therapeutic uses of hydrosols.

Eight Popular Hydrosols

Here are Suzanne Catty's notes on eight popular hydrosols (reprinted with permission):

Roman chamomile: Number one remedy for baby care, reduces teething pain and inflammation, calms diarrhea, promotes sleep, may be used as an eyewash or compress for conjunctivitis, calms sensitive skin, soothes burns and other skin irritations, mildly astringent, gently uplifting, recommended for stress.

Geranium/rose geranium: Great for skin care, balancing for all skin types, mild anti-inflammatory, promotes healing, balances male and female energies, lovely aroma.

Lavender: All-purpose, soothing on damaged or fragile skin, antiseptic, toner for all skin types, calms burns and abrasions, a great balancer for mind, body, and spirit.

Lemon verbena: General system tonic, anti-inflammatory, balancing and calming for hormones, skin toner, calms nerves and stage-fright, highly energetic, complex citrus aroma, delicate flavor.

Orange blossom/orange flower/neroli: Antistress, antispasmodic, can calm hysterics, excellent for delicate, sensitive skin and oily skin, very astringent, superb toner, clears skin irritations, lovely cologne or environmental spray.

Rose: Divine fragrance, treats dry or sensitive skin, highly energetic, promotes emotional balance, helps resolve blocks, deodorizes.

Rosemary: Mental and physical stimulant, digestive aid, antioxidant, great in hair products, toner for oily to normal skin, mild circulatory stimulant, compress for nerve pain, not for use during pregnancy, strong taste.

Witch hazel: Powerful anti-inflammatory, effective antiseptic, antifungal, anti-infectious, very strong antioxidant, free radical scavenger, may be used in antiaging treatments. Very different aroma from commercial witch hazel.

How to Use Hydrosols

- Spray hydrosols into the air to lift the spirits, increase energy, focus attention, deodorize, disinfect, and as an all-purpose air spray.
- Spray hydrosols onto sheets, blankets, and pillowcases for a fresh scent and to enhance sleep. Spray on towels, washcloths, shower curtains, and bath mats to deodorize bathrooms. Spray on cat litter boxes, too.
- For bath use, add 1 cup hydrosol (or more) to the tub. For children, use 1 teaspoon hydrosol for each year of age. For infants, use 1 teaspoon hydrosol per bath.
- Hydrosols tone the skin, moisturize, act as an aftershave lotion, and set makeup. Spray on the hair between shampoos or to help with styling.
- Add hydrosols to tea water and drinking water, using 2 tablespoons per quart, or as much as desired. For children, use 1 teaspoon per quart, and for infants, add 1 to 4 drops to each ½ cup of fluid.
- To use as a mouthwash, dilute 1 part hydrosol in 4 parts water, or use full-strength. For children, dilute 1 part hydrosol in 10 parts water.
- To use as a compress, add 3 to 5 tablespoons hydrosol to 1 quart cold water, saturate a washcloth or other fabric, and apply where needed. For children, use 2 to 3 teaspoons per quart of water.

"Sterilize application bottles before filling them, and store hydrosols in the coolest, darkest part of your house or in the refrigerator."

Discard any hydrosol that has an "off" odor or contains particulate matter. Bacteria can cause a hydrosol to "bloom" or spoil, and spoiled hydrosols can be harmful.

Hydrosols, says Catty, are thirty times more concentrated than a standard cup of tea. Diluted with water, tea, aloe vera juice or gel, or any other liquid, they can be used as medicinal-strength herbal teas. Left full strength, they can be used like diluted essential oils.

CHAPTER SEVEN

Detoxification

TODAY PEOPLE LIVE WITH SOMETHING unknown to thousands of generations of human ancestors. Our daily exposure to automobile exhaust, industrial and agricultural chemicals, and other sources of environmental pollution strain the body's filters and immune system.

There is much misunderstanding about detoxification. Most health enthusiasts think of detoxification as a specific program of herbs or supplements undertaken to remove impurities from the system.

In fact, detoxification goes on constantly as the body breaks down and removes waste products. If the body receives the nutrients it needs to perform this function well, it maintains itself in a state of health. If the process is impaired, health suffers. Unfortunately, most American bodies are overwhelmed with the burden of detoxification.

During the first stage of detoxification, the body identifies and separates waste products, toxins, and anything else that it doesn't need from the blood and lymph. Water-soluble material that can be excreted goes to the kidneys. Dehydration complicates the detoxification process, which is why consuming clean drinking water is so important. Anyone who is recovering from an illness, experiencing weight loss, changing to a natural diet, eliminating intestinal parasites, or recovering from treatment with conventional drugs should drink extra water throughout the day.

In Phase I of detoxification, waste products are made water-soluble and sent to the kidneys for elimination. The liver uses antioxidants and key minerals such as vitamins A, C, and E, bioflavonoids, selenium, copper, superoxide dismutase (SOD), zinc, and manganese during this phase. In Phase II, the liver needs glucuronic acid, sulfates from glutathione, acetyl-cysteine, and the amino acids taurine, arginine, ornithine, glutamine, glycine, and cysteine.

When someone is deficient in either Phase I or Phase II nutrients, backups and spillovers of waste products occur. Partially processed toxins traveling through the bloodstream may find a home in fatty tissue, or they may stay in the blood, infect healthy tissue, and cause new illnesses. Mitochondria are energy production units in the cells, and they are several times more sensitive to the presence of toxins and the lack of key nutrients than are normal cells. Mitochondria need vitamins E, K, and B-complex, niacin, coenzyme Q10, and the amino acid carnitine. A lack of nutritional support for mitochondria contributes to the overwhelming fatigue associated with rapid detoxification.

A diet of fresh, whole foods that contains high-quality protein, saturated and unsaturated fats, a variety of fresh fruits and vegetables, and sprouted grains provides all the fuel the liver and other organs need for efficient detoxification. Whole-food supplements such as those produced by Wysong and Standard Process help prevent any vitamin or mineral deficiency. Seacure (see page 104), is a whole-food source of amino acids. Colostrum and lactoferrin, described on page 112, support detoxification, and so do digestive enzymes taken between meals as described on page 91.

Milk thistle seed (*Silybum marianum*) regenerates the liver even in cases of hepatitis, exposure to environmental toxins, damage caused by pharmaceutical drugs, and mushroom poisoning. Therapeutic doses during detoxification can be much higher than label directions, such as 8 or more capsules or 2 tablespoons of tincture per day for a week or more as needed.

Aloe vera juice or gel helps remove toxins from the system while soothing the digestive tract. Daily doses of 1 to 2 tablespoons three times per day (use half this amount if the product is concentrated) protect the system from a variety of harmful compounds. During times of rapid detoxification, double the dosage of aloe vera.

Herbal Melange, a mudlike concentrate from Austrian peat moors that contains traces of hundreds of different plant species, is a traditional folk remedy with a worldwide following. Extensive European research has shown that it stimulates digestion, absorbs gas, binds acid, lowers alcohol levels, reduces cholesterol, repels parasites, removes harmful bacteria and detoxifies the entire gastrointestinal system. Take 1 teaspoon to 1 tablespoon in water between meals, twice or three times per day.

Essiac tea, which contains sheep sorrel, burdock root, slippery elm bark, and Turkey rhubarb root, is recommended by holistic health care practitioners for the treatment of tumors, thyroid disorders, skin conditions, and as a general health tonic. Because it supports the liver, its daily use helps maintain efficient detoxification. Burdock root is a tonic herb classified as an alterative, also known as a blood-cleansing herb. Slippery elm bark is a soothing, nutritive, demulcent herb which helps prevent irritation while enhancing digestion.

Some suggest that Essiac not be used by those with kidney disease or arthritis because of the oxalic acid in sheep sorrel and Turkey rhubarb root, although the blend has nonetheless helped many with these disorders. Turkey rhubarb root is not recommended for pregnant women.

Bupleurum, a Chinese herb sold in preparations such as Minor Bupleurum Formula, is exceptionally effective in the treatment of hepatitis, liver cancer, other diseases of the liver, and for detoxification support. Bupleurum preparations are sold in herb shops and health food stores that carry Chinese herbs, in Chinese markets, and by mail.

Maitake, reishi, shiitake, and several other medicinal mushrooms have received much publicity in recent years for their immune-stimulating properties. Any combination of medicinal mushrooms can be given with food or between meals to support efficient detoxification or for the prevention and treatment of all liver diseases, including hepatitis.

Citrus Pectin is a mucilaginous, water-soluble substance that attracts and holds liquid, swelling to form a viscous, glutinous mass. Clinical studies indicate that modified citrus pectin is absorbed into the bloodstream, where it attaches itself to unhealthy or undesirable cells, helping to remove them from the body.

Willard Water, described on page 110, improves digestion and the assimilation of nutrients, helps prevent stress caused by detoxification, aids in recovery from diseasse, and increases the effectiveness of herbs and nutritional supplements.

Wheat grass juice, powdered wheat grass, and other cereal grasses such as barley, oat, kamut, spelt, and rye grass, as well as green foods such as spirulina, chlorella, buckwheat lettuce, and sunflower seed sprouts, help prevent toxic reactions and rid the body of heavy metals, harmful chemicals, and other poisons. Use wheat grass juice and other grass juices sparingly as these are powerful medicines.

The common culinary herb cilantro, also known as Chinese parsley or coriander leaf, can accelerate the excretion of mercury from the body. A Japanese researcher discovered this by accident when mercury levels in the urine of a patient being tested for toxic metals increased after the patient consumed a Vietnamese soup containing cilantro. This led to several experiments, including one in which three mercury amalgam fillings were removed from a patient who had absorbed significant amounts of mercury. Without the use of chelation agents, daily consumption of cilantro removed the mercury within three weeks. Fresh cilantro can be substituted for basil in pesto recipes, added to soups, and used in Mexican dishes. A teaspoon of fresh minced or pureed cilantro per day is recommended after dental work and as part of any detoxification therapy.

Some products sold as detoxifying teas and diet aids have potentially serious side effects. For example, some popular diet teas and capsules contain stimulant herbs such as Ma huang (ephedra), caffeine-rich herbs such as kola nut or guarana, diuretic herbs such as juniper berry or buchu, disinfecting herbs such as uva ursi, and laxative herbs such as cascara sagrada or senna leaf. All of these are useful and effective when used appropriately, but they don't belong in herbal tea blends sold to the public for weight loss or detoxification, especially with vague labels that encourage their frequent or daily consumption. Some of these herbs are ingredients in well-designed herbal cleansing products, in which case they are combined with other plants that help balance their action, but to rely on ephedra, caffeine, and laxative or diuretic herbs to speed the metabolism, suppress the appetite, and cause rapid weight loss, is potentially dangerous.

Many herbal teas with "detox" in their names are more gentle and appropriate for daily use. But whether they come from the Ayurvedic practices of ancient India, European herbology,

Chinese medicine, or other traditions, these teas work best in combination with fresh fruits and vegetables, gentle sources of dietary fiber, and "green" foods.

CASTOR OIL PACKS

The castor oil pack is a type of fomentation or hot compress, only instead of using an herbal tea, it uses pharmaceutical grade castor oil, which can be purchased in drug and health food stores. Many herbalists, naturopaths, and other holistic health professionals use castor oil packs as a specific therapy for the liver. The procedure is simple, and though it's time consuming, it's relaxing. More important, castor oil packs help strengthen and heal not only the liver but other systems as well.

Saturate with castor oil a thick wool or cotton flannel two to eight layers thick, measuring 10 by 14 inches or larger when folded. Place it on the abdomen, especially over the liver area, cover with a plastic bag to keep things tidy (it helps to lie on a large towel while doing this), and top with a heating pad or hot water bottle. Lie still and let the pack heat up and stay hot for an hour. Wipe off the residue, place the oil-saturated pack in a resealable plastic storage bag. The saturated flannel can be reused for months and does not require refrigeration.

Castor oil packs have been shown in clinical use to improve elimination in the gastrointestinal and genitourinary tracts; stimulate peristalsis; maintain the mucous-membrane lining; improve assimilation; balance acid secretion in the stomach; stimulate liver, pancreas, and gall bladder secretions; improve the functioning of major organs, glands, and systems; stimulate the nervous system;

regulate metabolism; improve lymphatic circulation; and draw acids and infections from the body.

Some experts recommend the use of castor oil packs every other day for one or two weeks, then twice per week as needed. However, any schedule will produce good results, so "use as desired" is an appropriate instruction.

FOOD POISONING

Although the United States has one of the world's safest food supplies, a 1999 report from the federal government estimated that 76 million Americans suffer from food poisoning each year and approximately five thousand die from it. The herbs and supplements described here help treat most types of food poisoning.

The leading causes of food poisoning in the United States are campylobacter, salmonella, botulism, *Escherichia coli*, and *Listeria*.

Campylobacter is a bacteria commonly found in poultry and contaminated water. It is a leading cause of traveler's discomfort. Its symptoms, which include stomach cramps, diarrhea, chills, a high fever, headache, nausea, and vomiting, usually begin two to five days after eating contaminated chicken or other fowl. Most cases improve on their own. To help prevent the spread of campylobacter, cook poultry well, wash your hands after touching raw chicken, use separate cutting boards for meats and produce, and keep kitchen surfaces clean. Campylobacter found in poultry, cattle, and sheep cause similar symptoms two to five days after eating. In addition, blood may appear in the stool. Symptoms can last up to ten days.

Salmonella is a bacteria often found in chicken, eggs, meats, and raw milk. Its symptoms, which include stomach cramps, diarrhea, chills, a high fever, headache, nausea, and vomiting, usually develop quickly after contact with contaminated food. Most people who become ill from salmonella improve on their own within twenty-four hours. To help prevent the spread of salmonella, avoid food containing raw eggs unless you know the eggs are safe, use different utensils to handle raw and cooked food, and practice good hygiene. Salmonella is uncommon in healthy, organically raised, free-range chickens and their eggs. Some commercially raised sprouts have been infected with salmonella, but this is not a widespread problem.

Botulism is a deadly toxin produced by the spores of the bacteria *Clostridium botulinum*, which thrives in alkaline conditions away from oxygen. Botulism is usually associated with improperly preserved food, but in recent years it was discovered in blends of garlic and olive oil that were left at room temperature for several days. As a result, the FDA issued guidelines for the manufacture of salad dressings and flavored oils. Products containing garlic and vegetable oil must be processed at high temperature and pressure or acidified with lemon juice or vinegar to prevent botulism contamination. Although honey does not cause botulism in children or adults, infants are at risk, so honey is not recommended for infants. Botulism symptoms, which take between twenty-four to thirty-six hours to develop, include headache, dizziness, double vision, muscle paralysis, vomiting, impaired breathing, and difficulty swallowing. It is important to seek medical attention immediately because botulism can be fatal. Never eat food from cans or bottles that are punctured, cracked, bulging, rusted, sticky, or improperly sealed. Freezing, drying, and heating foods to 176 degrees Fahrenheit for twenty minutes or 194 degrees Fahrenheit for ten minutes helps destroy botulism spores.

Escherichia coli (*E. coli*) bacteria live in the intestines of humans and other animals, and they can contaminate meat, fruit, vegetables, or drinking water. In healthy humans, hydrochloric acid, digestive enzymes, and beneficial bacteria break down the *E. coli* and render it harmless, but under the right conditions in children, the elderly, and those with compromised immune systems, *E. coli* can be deadly. Symptoms include extremely painful stomach cramps, fever, and chills. These symptoms usually disappear in five to ten days, but the infection can lead to kidney failure and seizures in rare cases.

Listeria bacteria infect warmblooded animals, both wild and domestic. When transmitted to humans, *Listeria* usually causes flulike symptoms, but in those with weakened immune systems, it can cause meningitis and blood clotting. Occasionally *Listeria* is blamed for outbreaks of food poisoning, such as when hot dogs were recalled from New York markets after two people died.

Staphylococcus produces a toxin that can contaminate meat, poultry, egg products, tuna, potato salad, pasta salad, and cream-filled pastries. Its symptoms, which occur half an hour to eight hours after eating, include diarrhea, nausea, abdominal cramps, and vomiting.

Perfringens are bacteria in meat and meat products that survive cooking and reproduce after food cools and during storage. This type of food poisoning is most serious in the elderly. Its symptoms are mild nausea and vomiting that last less than a day.

Giardiasis is caused by *Giardia lamblia*, a parasite that contaminates some water supplies and is transferred to foods grown in or rinsed with contaminated water. Giardiasis is a common problem among hikers and campers because it infects most of the lakes and ponds in North America. Symptoms, which occur within one to three weeks of exposure, include diarrhea, constipation, severe cramping, abdominal pain, flatulence, loss of appetite, nausea, and vomiting.

Every year news stories describe food-poisoning breakouts at state fairs, restaurants, and family gatherings. According to public health officials, most cases of food poisoning don't make headlines because they are never reported. In fact, many victims of food poisoning never make the connection between what they ate and how they feel, mistaking the symptoms of bacterial contamination for the flu or a virus. Most cases of food-caused illness in the home can be traced to careless hygiene and the incomplete cooking of contaminated meat, poultry, and eggs, and they can be prevented with common sense and the frequent use of soap and water.

In every outbreak of food poisoning, some people develop only mild symptoms while others become seriously ill. Children are usually at greater risk, and children who recently took antibiotics are at greatest risk. In outbreaks that resulted in death, most or all of the children who died had recently been treated with antibiotics. In addition to avoiding antibiotics except in emergencies, it is important to restore the beneficial intestinal bacteria antibiotics destroy as described on page 61.

Like beneficial bacteria in the intestines, hydrochloric acid in the stomach kills harmful bacteria. For those with insufficient HCl levels, taking this supplement with meals helps protect against food poisoning.

CHAPTER EIGHT

Treating Digestive Disorders

THE CAUSE OF MOST DIGESTIVE problems is diet, described in detail in this book's first four chapters. Eating the foods that are right for you, and staying away from those that are wrong for you, is the most important step you can take toward reversing and curing digestive disorders.

In addition, here are some drug-free ways to treat and prevent common problems.

CELIAC DISEASE, CELIAC SPRUE
(See pages 54 to 56)

COLIC

Spasmodic abdominal pains in young infants and children, accompanied by irritability or crying, colic also refers to conditions of flatulence and other symptoms of indigestion in infants up to three months of age. Its causes include overfeeding, swallowing air, or emotional upset, but its primary cause is probably dietary. Cow's milk, soy, corn, wheat, and eggs are frequent offenders, while flatulence and gas can be caused by a nursing mother eating garlic, onion, beans, or cabbage.

For temporary relief from colic, Europe's favorite remedy is "gripe water," an old fashioned infusion of dill seed rarely used in the United States even though it's still listed in the United

States Pharmacopoeia. Make your own by pouring 1 cup boiling water over 1 to 2 teaspoons gently crushed seeds; cover and let stand until cool. Give in teaspoon doses until it brings relief. Chamomile, a more familiar herb, is the first choice of many herbalists for treating colic in infants and children. Like gripe water, chamomile tea can be given to infants and children by the teaspoon. Both teas are recommended to nursing mothers; drink up to three cups of medicinal-strength tea daily.

Chamomile, dill, or fennel hydrosol can be applied to an infant's stomach and administered orally. Suzanne Catty recommends adding 1 teaspoon hydrosol to 1 cup warm water for application to an infant's abdomen, and up to 3 drops hydrosol to ¼ cup fluid for oral consumption, but these three hydrosols are so safe and gentle—assuming they are fresh and of therapeutic quality—that they can be applied full-strength to the abdomen and dropped into a baby's mouth with an eyedropper, a few drops every ten minutes. Nursing mothers can add 1 tablespoon hydrosol to 1 pint (2 cups) drinking water or other liquids.

In *Essential Oils and Aromatherapy*, Dr. Valerie Worwood recommends massaging an infant's abdomen with 3 drops essential oil (1 drop each of Roman chamomile, lavender, and geranium) diluted in 2 tablespoons sweet almond oil or, for more serious cases, 1 drop dill essential oil diluted in 1 tablespoon almond oil.

CONSTIPATION

Sluggish, infrequent bowel movements are almost always caused by insufficient fiber in the diet, dehydration, and physical inactivity, though it is sometimes caused by drugs or a physical obstruction. Assuming you don't require surgical intervention, drink a large glass of water every hour or two all day long, stir 1 teaspoon to 1 tablespoon of psyllium husk powder, guar gum, pectin, or a similar soluble fiber into a glass of water every morning and night, and take a mild herbal laxative, such as a small amount of cascara sagrada or senna. Health food stores sell several products containing these herbs.

Prevent future constipation by eating more raw fruits and vegetables, whole grains, and other whole foods. Prunes and other dried fruit are known to have mild laxative properties.

Dilute 15 drops rosemary essential oil, 10 drops lemon, and 5 drops peppermint oil in 2 tablespoons carrier oil and massage the lower abdomen in a clockwise direction three times daily. Alternatively, use patchouli, cedarwood, or angelica essential oil.

DIARRHEA

Loose, watery stools can be caused by viral and bacterial infections, nervous excitement, food poisoning, parasites, or diseases of the digestive tract. A healthy system recovers quickly from brief episodes of diarrhea, but when prolonged, the dehydration and mineral imbalances diarrhea produces can be fatal.

Obviously, the symptom's cause must be addressed. If it's due to Crohn's disease, irritable bowel syndrome, or a similar digestive disorder, see pages 54 to 56.

Traveler's diarrhea can be prevented by taking herbs or supplements that kill viruses, bacteria, parasites, molds, fungi, and other microorganisms. Olive leaf extract, grapefruit seed extract, and bee propolis are examples.

To treat diarrhea, take 1 teaspoon to 1 tablespoon green clay, the kind sold in health food stores, stirred into a glass of water. Clay has a soothing effect on irritated intestinal lining; it absorbs toxins and helps reverse the condition. Arrowroot, Jerusalem artichoke flour, carob powder, and other starches help reduce the amount of fluid lost and restore intestinal flora. Small amounts of powdered psyllium husk, pectin, or other sources of soluble fiber have the same effect. All of these should be mixed with water rather than taken in capsules. Astringent teas such as bayberry, wild oak bark, blackberry leaf, or cranesbill; cayenne pepper in capsules; large amounts of acidophilus or similar supplements; and large quantities of water with a pinch of unrefined sea salt to prevent dehydration are all appropriate therapies. Blueberries and blackberries, especially blackberries, are so effective that some herbalists keep dried blackberries on hand to grind and mix with water as first-aid treatment. Even blackberry jam will help, they claim.

Pediatricians recommend electrolyte replacement formulas for infants and children with diarrhea, and some physicians tell adult patients to drink sports beverages to replace lost minerals. However, these products all contain refined table salt, artificial flavors, chemical preservatives, and in many cases artificial colors as well. You can prepare a much better product at home.

Electrolyte Replacement Formula

2   cups filtered or bottled water
1   tablespoon unrefined sea salt
¼   teaspoon liquid colloidal trace minerals
½   cup raw honey (for infants use ½ cup brown rice syrup
    or barley malt syrup instead of honey, as honey may
    cause botulism poisoning in infants)

If available, add 1 to 2 tablespoons therapeutic-quality Roman chamomile, German chamomile, or lavender hydrosol. These calming hydrosols have a soothing, restorative effect. Alternatively, brew chamomile tea and use it instead of water.

Powdered acidophilus can be added as well. Probiotic powders containing bifidus bacteria and other beneficial bacteria help restore the proper balance of intestinal flora.

To treat diarrhea in adults, Dr. Worwood recommends different essential oils depending on the cause of the problem. For diarrhea caused by food, she recommends massaging the entire abdomen with a blend of 3 drops peppermint, 2 drops chamomile, and 1 drop eucalyptus essential oil in 1 teaspoon carrier oil. For nervous diarrhea, use 3 drops lavender, 2 drops eucalyptus, and 1 drop chamomile in 1 teaspoon carrier oil. For diarrhea caused by viral infections, use 3 drops thyme, 2 drops lavender, and 1 drop tea tree oil in 1 teaspoon carrier oil. In addition, add 1 drop of peppermint (if food- or nerve-related) or eucalyptus (if virus-related) essential oil to 1 teaspoon honey; dilute in a glass of warm water, and sip slowly.

GAS, FLATULENCE

Intestinal gas or "wind" can be caused by eating too fast, swallowing air, eating gas-producing foods such as beans, drinking carbonated beverages, chewing gum, talking with your mouth full, or eating dairy products if you are lactose intolerant. In addition to the digestive enzymes Beano and Lactaid (see page 90), look to carminative herb teas for relief: angelica root, aniseed, caraway seed, cardamon seed, catnip, cayenne pepper, celery seed, chamomile, cinnamon, cloves, fennel seed, ginger, lemon balm, licorice root, peppermint, or spearmint. A strongly brewed lemon balm tea, for example, or a blend of ginger and licorice root tea is often very beneficial. In severe cases, take two capsules containing activated charcoal with a glass of water every twenty minutes until symptoms subside.

Hydrosols can be added to tea water. Fennel, bay leaf, lemon balm, and basil hydrosols help relieve gas and bloating. Add up to 2 tablespoons per quart of water or herbal tea.

The essential oils of cardamom, peppermint, coriander, dill, eucalyptus, or spearmint can be added to a carrier oil and massaged over the abdomen. Therapeutic-quality peppermint oil can be applied full-strength, 1 to 5 drops at a time, to the abdomen. In addition, a drop of any of these essential oils can be mixed with a teaspoon of honey and swallowed from the spoon or added to herbal tea.

Prevent flatulence by taking Swedish Bitters (see page 3) before eating, eating slowly, chewing food well, avoiding sources of swallowed air, avoiding foods that don't agree with you, taking hydrochloric acid supplements or digestive enzymes as needed, supplementing your diet with acidophilus and other friendly bacteria, and avoiding stress while eating.

HEARTBURN

Also known as gastroesophageal reflux disease (GERD), heartburn has nothing to do with the heart but was named for the approximate location of the burning pain that occurs when stomach acid leaks into the esophagus. This often happens when people overeat or eat foods that are too spicy or too greasy. Common offenders include chocolate, caffeine, onions, tomatoes, citrus fruits, and peppery sausages. A Mayo Clinic survey of 1,500 patients concluded that alcohol, smoking, aspirin, and nonsteroidal anti-inflammatory drugs, all of which are considered risk factors for gastroesophageal reflux disease, are in fact not important. The primary risk factor found in the survey was obesity.

To alleviate heartburn, drink an 8-ounce glass of water every twenty to thirty minutes until pain subsides, drink a cup of licorice root tea, or take 100 grams of deglycyrrhizinated licorice. Prevent this condition by eating small meals often rather than large meals infrequently, increase the time between eating dinner and lying down or going to bed, avoid or greatly reduce caffeine consumption, avoid foods that are overspiced, greasy, sugary, or acidic, take Swedish Bitters before and after eating, experiment with the basic rules of food combining, and take acidophilus daily.

Drugs that relax smooth muscles, such as the asthma drug theophylline, contribute to the problem because heartburn occurs when the esophageal sphincter muscle relaxes and allows stomach acid and pepsin to enter the esophagus. Peppermint has a similar effect, which is why peppermint is not recommended for heartburn.

HEMORRHOIDS

Hemorrhoids, or piles, are painful varicose veins in the rectum or anus. The most common cause is chronic constipation, often associated with a lack of exercise. They are also common during pregnancy.

To help relieve hemorrhoid symptoms, drink more water and

fluids, increase soluble and insoluble fiber in the diet, improve nutrition with raw juices and whole fruits and vegetables, take a tablespoon of cold-pressed vegetable oil daily, and move bowels promptly instead of suppressing their movements.

Apply aloe vera gel several times per day to soothe and cool inflamed tissue. Any strong astringent tea such as bayberry bark, witch hazel bark, wild oak bark, prince's pine, uva ursi, or cranesbill can be used as a compress. So can full-strength witch hazel hydrosol, which is very different from the drugstore witch hazel, or the hydrosols of neroli or cypress. According to hydrosol authority Suzanne Catty, all of these have an astringent as well as healing influence. Swedish Bitters can be diluted with an equal amount of water and used the same way. Soak a washcloth or cotton handkerchief with cold tea, hydrosol, or diluted Swedish bitters and apply to the affected area several times daily.

According to Kurt Schnaubelt, the essential oil of niaouli (*Melaleuca quinquenervia veridiflora,* MQV) from Madagascar has the ability to tighten tissue and is used for hemorrhoids. "The oil is effective for specific and general skin problems," he explains, "and can be used undiluted without risk." Apply it full-strength to a wet washcloth, 1 or 2 drops at a time, and hold to the affected area.

IRRITABLE BOWEL SYNDROME

Known as irritable bowel syndrome (IBS), irritable bowel disease (IBD), spastic colon, and irritable colon, this inconvenient disorder shares many symptoms with other inflammatory bowel diseases, including Crohn's disease and ulcerative colitis. All these conditions can produce stomach upsets, bloating, belching, flatulence, nausea, spasms causing diarrhea, periods of constipation, and, in the case of IBS, sharp and stabbing pain.

The restricted carbohydrate diet described on pages 54 to 56 reverses and in many cases cures these disorders. Several supplements described in chapter 4 help as well, including systemic oral enzyme therapy, acidophilus and other probiotic supplements, Seacure, and colostrum. In addition, herbs such as aloe vera, licorice root, and Swedish Bitters are helpful. If bouts of illness are triggered by intestinal parasites, see the recommendations for that condition on page 191.

In Europe, peppermint is widely used for stomach, liver, gallbladder, and pancreatic disturbances. Because the active menthol ingredients in peppermint are rapidly absorbed in the stomach and upper gastrointestinal tract, peppermint tea or tincture has little effect on the lower bowels. Enteric-coated peppermint oil capsules, which are sold in pharmacies, deliver peppermint's active ingredients to the colon. The dosage recommended for IBS patients is usually 2 to 3 capsules a day between meals. The only side effect noted has been a temporary burning sensation in the rectal area after a bowel movement, which is caused by excess, unabsorbed menthol. Reducing the dosage relieves this harmless side effect. Peppermint is not recommended for young children.

Daniel Penoel recommends the essential oil of tropical basil (*Ocimum basilicum, CT methyl chavicol*) for all types of intestinal cramping. Apply several drops to the abdomen and add a drop to honey as described above.

Suzanne Catty notes that fennel hydrosol calms stomachaches and is an antispasmodic with a special affinity for digestive conditions. Lemon balm (melissa) hydrosol is a calming digestive aid. These hydrosols can be applied to the abdomen as well as taken internally.

NAUSEA, MOTION SICKNESS

Motion sickness can interfere with all types of travel. Pregnancy brings bouts of morning sickness, and anyone can experience nausea from time to time.

One of the most effective nausea prevention herbs is ginger-root. Ginger ale, gingersnaps, and ginger candies are often recommended, but powdered ginger in capsules works more efficiently. For best results, take as many ginger capsules as needed to create a gentle heartburnlike reaction in the throat; start with 2 or 3, wait for five minutes, and increase as necessary. Some need as many as 8 or 10 to produce this effect. Take ginger fifteen to twenty minutes before leaving on a trip, and its beneficial effect should last for several hours. Repeat as needed.

One drop of peppermint essential oil applied to the back of the neck or tasted on the tongue is another effective treatment, though it is not recommended for children under age three, and for children under twelve the peppermint oil should be diluted in a teaspoon of honey. A drop of peppermint oil applied to a car's upholstery also helps prevent car sickness.

Basil hydrosol helps relieve nausea, especially stress-related nausea. Hydrosols can be sprayed into the air, into the mouth, and onto the skin, as well as added to tea and other beverages.

PARASITES

Intestinal worms cause a confusing variety of symptoms, from digestive distress to allergic and autoimmune reactions. Parasites that enter through the digestive tract usually cause changes in appetite, stomach and abdominal discomfort, bloating, nausea, flatulence, intestinal cramping, and diarrhea; they eventually lead to malabsorption syndrome and other chronic digestive problems. Eight out of ten people in North America harbor one or more parasites, and the rate is increasing. International travel, food and water contamination, household pets, and day-care centers all help spread parasites, and antibiotic drugs make people more susceptible by killing the beneficial intestinal bacteria that help prevent parasite infestation.

Acidophilus and other probiotic supplements will not kill parasites, but they strengthen the body's defenses against them. Raw garlic and garlic supplements help strip mucus from intestinal walls, making parasites more vulnerable to natural therapies. The proteolytic enzyme protease digests parasites if taken on an empty stomach between meals. For best results, take garlic with coarsely ground or well-chewed whole pumpkin seeds, which mechanically irritate internal parasites, then wait an hour before taking a supplement containing protease or pancreatic enzymes. The round black seeds of a fresh papaya contain the enzyme papain, which also helps remove parasites. Foods rich in soluble fiber such as ground flaxseed, shredded carrots, psyllium husks, agar-agar, comfrey root, citrus pectin, apple pectin, figs, prunes, dates, and papaya help expose parasites by removing the intestinal debris and mucus in which they hide, and by sweeping intestinal walls and stimulating elimination, they help remove weakened or damaged parasites.

Tapeworms, a common human parasite, are paralyzed by pelletierine, an alkaloid drug found in pomegranates. Whenever pomegranates are in season, eat several and follow them with dried fruit to help flush any incapacitated tapeworms from the body.

Many who have suffered from the debilitating cramping

caused by *Giardia lamblia,* a parasite that infects all of North America's lakes, say that the only product that immediately relieves its pain is aloe vera. Aloe vera doesn't kill parasites, but it is an excellent first-aid treatment for use with other herbs and, when needed, prescription drugs.

Check your health food store for herbal capsules or tinctures containing parasite-repelling herbs. One of the most popular antiparasite programs combines wormwood, cloves, and black walnut hulls, but there are many effective herbal products for preventing this widespread problem.

ULCERS

Ulcers have long been associated with "wrong" foods. For years, ulcer patients were told to stay away from spicy foods, especially cayenne pepper, and encouraged to eat bland foods, especially dairy products. Then researchers discovered that dairy products often worsen ulcers, while cayenne pepper stops internal bleeding and helps prevent its recurrence.

One of the most effective European ulcer remedies is fresh cabbage juice. One quart per day for a week literally cures most ulcers. Another popular herbal treatment is licorice root tea or extract. While it is unusual for whole-root licorice tea to cause side effects, the glycyrrhizic acid in concentrated European extracts caused fluid retention and elevated blood pressure in long-term users. To prevent these problems, deglycyrrhizinated licorice (DGL) products were developed, some of which are sold in American pharmacies as over-the-counter remedies for indigestion. In addition, 2 ounces of aloe vera gel or juice taken three times daily is recommended for ulcer pain.

Mastic or gum mastic, the resin or pitch of a Mediterranean tree, was treasured by the ancient Greeks, Romans, and Arabs as a digestive aid. Known as the original chewing gum, mastic improves the breath, treats and prevents tooth and gum disease, and relieves indigestion. Now mastic is becoming famous as an ulcer cure.

The spiral-shaped bacteria *Heliobacter pylori*, which infects an estimated 50 percent of the world's population, has been shown to cause gastritis, an inflammation of the stomach lining, which in turn causes digestive complaints including discomfort, bloating, nausea, and the formation of ulcers. Some researchers suspect it may cause stomach cancer as well. *H. pylori* survives below the mucous membranes of the stomach and duodenum. Nearly all duodenal ulcer patients are infected with the bacteria, as are an estimated 70 percent of those with gastric ulcers. Gastric cancers occur in patients who have *H. pylori* infections or who have had them in the past.

In research reported in *The New England Journal of Medicine* and other medical journals, Farhad U. Huwez, Ph.D., found that mastic killed seven strains of *H. pylori*, even those that are resistant to prescription drugs, by inducing fatal structural changes in the organism. Low doses of mastic, such as 1 to 2 grams per day (the amounts traditionally used in foods) can cure peptic ulcers within two weeks. Because it kills *E. coli*, salmonella, and other harmful bacteria, mastic has also been used as an antidote for food poisoning. Unprocessed mastic "pearls" can be chewed with food, or the resin can be taken in capsules (see Resources).

Bee propolis, described on page 107, is an effective ulcer therapy. Another is manuka honey. The manuka, a small shrubby bush that grows only in New Zealand, is sometimes called the New Zealand tea tree. According to researchers at the University of

Waikato in New Zealand, manuka honey contains hydrogen per-oxide and traces of antibacterial substances from plant nectar. The *H. pylori* bacteria seems to be five to ten times more sensitive to manuka honey than any other honey. In New Zealand honey, the level of antibacterial activity is measured on a scale of 1 to 15 indicating the Unique Manuka Factor, or UMF. A level of 10 or more indicates significant antibacterial activity.

CHAPTER NINE

Arthritis, Rheumatism, and Joint Pain

THE ILLNESSES ASSOCIATED WITH inflammation are both different and similar. Rheumatoid arthritis is an autoimmune disease, osteoarthritis is the degeneration of weight-bearing joints, gout is caused by the buildup of uric acid in the body, fibromyalgia (also called fibrositis) and lupus are inflammations of connective tissue, bursitis involves small sacs of fibrous tissue filled with fluid, and ankylosing spondylitis is a rheumatic disease of the backbone that can fuse joints. Their definitions and diagnoses vary, but all these illnesses produce the same debilitating pain that prevents people from moving freely and living a full, active, happy life.

Of all the "natural" approaches to the treatment of arthritis and other inflammatory illnesses, the most widely used is diet. Although most American physicians still discount their patients' observations that certain foods seem to cause swelling and inflammation, American researchers have begun to confirm what is common medical knowledge in other countries.

In studies reported in the *British Medical Journal, Clinical Rheumatology, Arthritis and Rheumatism, Annals of Internal Medicine, The Lancet,* and other leading medical journals, physicians have measured significant joint swelling (as much as two ring sizes in fingers), pain, loss of grip strength, reduced range of motion, and other symptoms of inflammation within hours of the patient's consumption of key foods. Several tests were double-blind, placebo-controlled clinical trials.

When patients with osteoarthritis and rheumatoid arthritis are placed on medically supervised fasts, their symptoms disappear. This is such a common reaction that researchers often recommend short-term fasting for rapid pain relief and temporary remission of nearly all arthritic conditions. Figuring out which foods to eat when it's time to end the fast is the challenge. Some nutritionists who supervise fasting patients test them with foods hidden in capsules; others reintroduce one food at a time (such as one food per meal or one per day) until something triggers arthritis symptoms. Another approach is to eliminate common allergens such as wheat and dairy products and observe the result. The connections between diet and inflammatory illnesses are so well established that anyone can explore them and expect at least partial relief.

Some experts say that arthritis is a cooked food disease and that increasing the amount of raw food in the diet to at least 70 or 75 percent successfully treats arthritis. This therapy is popular in health spas in Europe and North America. The restricted carbohydrate diet described on pages 54 to 56 and its counterparts have worked well for many with arthritis, but so have diets that restrict or eliminate animal protein. Every expert seems to have a different list of "most offending" foods. Restrictive diets are never easy, especially when they deviate from the social norm, and experimenting to find the foods your body reacts to takes time and effort, but freedom from pain and inflammation is a powerful incentive. Discovering one's best foods and consuming them raw whenever possible and always whole rather than refined or processed is an important strategy.

One connection between joint pain and diet is obvious: most arthritis patients are overweight. Excess weight puts increased stress on weight-bearing joints such as knees and ankles, making movement even more painful than it would be otherwise. It is difficult for anyone on America's refined-food diet to lose weight even if they are physically active. Add the sedentary lifestyle that accompanies the pain of arthritis and losing weight is almost impossible. But when someone with an inflammatory disease makes significant dietary changes, both excess weight and joint pain can disappear.

BEST-SELLING ARTHRITIS SUPPLEMENTS

Among arthritis patients, glucosamine and chondroitin sulfate have become popular supplements. However, these isolated nutrients represent less than 2 percent of the nutritional elements in connective tissue, all of which are vital to the health of joint cartilage, intervertebral discs, and vascular walls. Chondroitin sulfate is a mucopolysaccharide (complex molecule) that gives elasticity and spongelike shock-absorbing properties to the joints; glucosamine, the amino sugar of glucose, is a component of mucopolysaccharides and glycoproteins in connective tissue.

In contrast, supplements made from cold-sterilized, organically raised cattle and poultry bones contain over a hundred nutritional elements that are needed for healthy joints. The Wysong product Contifin contains a spectrum of collagen types (I–IX), proteoglycans, and glycosaminogyclans, including chondroitin, glucosamine, hyaluronan, keratan, dermatan, heparan, heparin, hyaluronic acid, decorin, giblycan, and fibromodulin. Standard Process makes several similar products, which strengthen the teeth and bones as well as joints and connective tissue. Several companies make supplements from bone-source microcrystalline hydroxyappatite (calcium orthophosphate), another recommended ingredient.

The supplement MSM, which stands for methylsufonylmethane, is a source of nutritional sulfur credited for improving many disorders, including arthritis. Sulfur is essential for healthy cells throughout the body, especially in the bones, joints, and skin. But raw foods contain significant quantities of MSM, and some vegetables, such as garlic, are exceptionally high in sulfur. Fresh raw garlic and supplements made from fermented garlic, such as Kyolic brand extract, have therapeutic benefits that go beyond those of a synthetic supplement such as MSM.

According to Jonathan Wright, M.D., MSM taken for several months or more can strip the trace mineral molybdenum from the body. He recommends taking a small amount of molybdenum (50 to 150 micrograms daily) to compensate.

ENZYME THERAPY

In the 1940s, English rheumatic researcher Arnold Renshaw, M.D., conducted four to six autopsies daily for several years. A high incidence of intestinal atrophy and deformation in the bodies he examined, especially in the small intestine, led him to speculate that rheumatoid arthritis might be a deficiency disease stemming from an enzyme deficiency that interferes with protein digestion and metabolism balance.

Renshaw tested his theory using a dried enzyme extract of intestinal mucosa prepared by a pharmaceutical company. Rheumatic patients took the enzyme in capsules after meals. In seven years, over 700 patients were tested, and good results were obtained in cases of rheumatoid arthritis, osteoarthritis, fibromyalgia (fibrositis), ankylosing spondylitis, and Still's disease, a joint disease affecting children. In a series of 556 cases of various types, 283 were found to be much improved and 219 somewhat improved; of 292 cases of rheumatoid arthritis, 264 showed improvement. Most patients responded slowly, requiring several months to achieve results, especially when the illness had already lasted for years. In some cases, between one and two years of daily enzyme supplementation were needed before blood tests showed normal sedimentation.

Edward Howell, M.D., studied food enzymes and human health for more than fifty years, and his book *Enzyme Nutrition: The Food Enzyme Concept* describes much of the research conducted on these important catalysts. Even Howell's worst cases of longstanding osteoarthritis and rheumatoid arthritis showed improvement, though the therapy worked slowly, often requiring months of daily supplementation or adherance to an all-raw vegetarian diet.

Systemic oral enzyme therapy (see page 91), in which digestive enzymes are taken between meals on an empty stomach, is a popular European treatment for arthritis, rheumatism, and related disorders. In addition, insufficient hydrochloric acid leads to the incomplete digestion of proteins and fats, which results in inflammation. See pages 86 to 88 for information about HCl supplements.

ENVIRONMENTAL CAUSES

Can arthritis and other rheumatic illnesses be caused by environmental allergies? The first physician to suggest a connection was Theron Randolph, M.D., the founder of environmental medicine. After testing over a thousand arthritics, Dr. Randolph found significant links between their arthritis and their reactions to foods, chemicals, perfumes, tobacco, and other substances.

According to Marshall Mandell, M.D., director of the New England Foundation for Allergic and Environmental Diseases, "Allergies may or may not cause arthritis, but they definitely play a major role in a majority of cases because they often aggravate and perpetuate the condition." When allergic substances are eliminated, avoided, or contacted less frequently, the arthritis is usually relieved or eliminated. In tests of over six thousand patients, Mandell found that foods, chemicals, grasses, pollen, molds, and other airborne substances caused allergic reactions in the joints of nearly 85 percent of the arthritics he tested. Other studies have shown that food additives, bacteria, yeasts, fungi, and protozoa can trigger or aggravate arthritic symptoms.

One way to identify possible allergens is to isolate the patient in a "clean" (allergy-free) environment for five days during which the patient consumes nothing but untreated, uncontaminated spring water. Foods and chemicals are introduced one at a time and the patient's reaction is carefully monitored. Knowing what chemicals or conditions to avoid has lessened the arthritic symptoms of many who have undergone this analysis.

MALILLUMINATION

In addition to eating the wrong foods and digesting them poorly, arthritis patients are light-deprived. Spending most of their time indoors, avoiding the sun, and protecting their eyes with sunglasses, they suffer from malillumination. As John Ott discovered (see pages 16 to 18), the simplest cure for arthritis and other bone and joint disorders is daily exposure to unfiltered natural light.

Anything that interferes with the transmission of unfiltered natural light contributes to malillumination, including glass windows and windshields, contact lenses, and eyeglasses. The endocrine system needs full-spectrum natural light. The only source of this essential nutrient is found outdoors; not even full-spectrum light bulbs provide it.

HERBS AND ESSENTIAL OILS

Many herbal teas, capsules, and tinctures are traditional arthritis therapies, among them alfalfa; blue-red berries (cherries are by themselves an effective gout treatment); boswellia, the resin of a tree from India; devil's claw, the root of an African herb, which is popular in Europe; feverfew, an herb that prevents migraine headaches as well as relieving joint pain; ginger, the familiar culinary herb; horsetail, which is unusually rich in the joint-repairing mineral silica; turmeric, the yellow spice used in curry powder; and white willow bark, the "original" aspirin.

In their book *Beyond Aspirin*, Thomas M. Newmark and Paul Schulick explain that excessive inflammation is caused by by-products of the enzyme cycloxygenase-2, or COX-2. Many herbs, such as most of those listed above, contain COX-2 inhibitors, which gives them anti-inflammatory properties.

Some of the most effective over-the-counter creams and liniments for the relief of arthritis contain capsaicin, the ingredient that makes cayenne pepper hot. Capsaicin's pain relief is cumulative; that is, the more often it is applied, the more effectively it works. However, those who are sensitive to foods in the night-shade family, which include peppers, may not be able to use these products.

Dozens of essential oils are used in massage blends that treat osteoarthritis, rheumatism, gout, and related diseases. Valerie Ann Worwood's three-stage protocol begins with daily baths using a blend of 30 drops fennel, 16 drops cypress, and 10 drops juniper essential oil; for each bath, mix 3 cups Epsom salts, 1 cup rock salt, and 4 drops of the essential oil blend. After two weeks of daily baths, the patient is ready for the second stage of baths and massages with different essential oil blends depending on the type of arthritis; a third stage, which involves using still different essential oils, completes the therapy.

Kurt Schnaubelt considers the essential oil of the Italian ever-lasting (*Helichrysum italicum*) an important anti-inflammatory and cell-regenerating agent. "The pain-reducing, analgesic, and regen-erative effect of everlasting is unique," he explains. "If applied in time [after injury], it prevents hemorrhaging. It is very effective for joint pain associated with rheumatoid arthritis." He recom-mends yarrow essential oil as an anti-inflammatory for neuralgia or tendinitis. Therapeutic-quality helichrysum or yarrow oil can be applied full-strength to wet skin as described on page 159, or it can be added to a carrier oil. Massage-oil blends containing jo-joba and castor oil work especially well for arthritis because they are absorbed more quickly and deeply than other oils.

Hydrosols can be sprayed full-strength on painful joints, ap-plied as soothing compresses, added to drinking water and herbal teas, and added to bathwater to soothe aches and pains. Suzanne Catty notes that juniper hydrosol eases rheumatic and arthritic pain, as does balsam fir hydrosol, which has a wonder-ful, woodsy taste and fragrance.

GOUT

Gout is an illness that, although different from arthritis, causes similar symptoms: joint inflammation, acute pain, swelling, redness, and heat. Gout attacks can occur without warning, resolve within a few days or weeks, and recur after pain-free periods that last months or years. Although many different joints may be affected, gout most often affects the big toe, causing it to become swollen and inflamed. Other gout-affected joints include the knees, thumbs, and elbows. Gout attacks may be accompanied by fever and fatigue.

Initial gout attacks usually strike at night and are preceded by a specific event, such as excessive alcohol consumption, trauma, certain drugs, or surgery. Other triggers include stress, infection, fad diets that result in rapid weight loss, and the development of illnesses that increase uric acid production, such as psoriasis, cancer, and some blood disorders. Excess weight, high blood fat levels, and diabetes also increase the incidence of gout. Although most patients experience another attack within one year of the first, nearly 7 percent of gout sufferers never have a second attack. The condition affects approximately three out of every thousand adults, and 95 percent affected are men over the age of thirty.

Unlike arthritis, gout has a single chemical cause, an overabundance of uric acid crystals in the joints, the jagged edges of which irritate tissue and cause pain and inflammation. Uric acid is a by-product of protein metabolism of the liver. High uric acid levels in the blood mark the first stages of gout, even if symptoms have not yet materialized. Chronic gout usually follows years of crystalline deposit formation in joints and cartilage, including cartilage of the ear.

Some experts associate the development of gout with abscessed teeth or chronically infected tonsils, both of which slowly release toxins into the bloodstream, and many gout sufferers had excessive nosebleeds and dry eczema on the knee in childhood. In the elderly, gout may affect many joints simultaneously, including those not usually associated with the disease. Although gout runs in families and a susceptibility to gout may be genetic, diet plays a key role in its development.

Gout has always been associated with rich living. Cartoons from the eighteenth and nineteenth centuries show gout victims as overweight, fashionably dressed men surrounded by wine and fatty foods, feet resting on elevated cushions, scowling in pain at their throbbing big toes. Animal protein, rich fatty foods, and alcohol are the primary causes of gout because these foods contain purine, which promotes the production of uric acid. Other sources of purine are fungi and yeasts that contaminate foods or take up residence in the body. Gout's connection to fungi and to candida yeast infections explains why vegetarians who eat foods containing yeast, white flour, and sugar can develop gout as easily as carnivores do.

Another underlying cause, according to Jonathan Wright, M.D., is the fructose added to processed foods. Fructose can raise blood uric acid, he warns, so gout patients should avoid foods that contain fructose, corn syrup, and high-fructose corn syrup. Whole fruit itself does not seem to be a problem.

Food sources of purine include red meats, shellfish, anchovies, herring, sardines, mussels, all organ meats, asparagus, and yeast products, including brewer's yeast, nutritional yeast, and baker's yeast. Anti-gout diets eliminate the consumption of purine-rich foods as well as coffee and other sources of caffeine, sugar, refined carbohydrates, most commercially prepared foods, saturated fats, margarine, shortening, commercial salad dressings, protein supplements, and lentils. Alcohol increases uric acid levels by accelerating purine metabolism and impairing kidney function.

Essential fatty acids such as those found in the oil of flax, borage, and evening primrose seeds help relieve the inflammation of this disease. However, the deep-sea fish oils that have been shown to reduce the inflammation of arthritis are likely to exacerbate gout. Whole grains, especially sprouted grains, are important because their pantothenic acid converts uric acid to urea and ammonia, but for best results, avoid bread, and consume dishes made from grain that has been soaked for several hours before cooking.

The most helpful vitamin supplements for gout patients are folic acid, which inhibits an enzyme essential for uric acid production, and pantothenic acid, which breaks down uric acid. Whole-food B-complex supplements provide both nutrients. Large doses of synthetic niacin (vitamin B_3) can elevate uric acid and should be avoided. There may be a link between vitamin A toxicity and gout, a good reason to focus on food sources of vitamin A, such as carrot juice, rather than megavitamin supplements. Vitamin C increases uric acid excretion and lowers blood uric acid; food-source supplements contain the entire vitamin C complex while avoiding problems caused by synthetic vitamin C (ascorbic acid).

In addition to drinking between two and four quarts of water daily, which keeps the urine diluted and promotes the excretion of uric acid, gout patients benefit from drinking freshly prepared raw juices. Some popular recipes for relief from gout contain equal parts of carrots and spinach, carrots with beets and cucumbers, carrots with beets and coconut, or carrots with celery, spinach, and parsley.

Cherries, bilberries, hawthorn berries, blueberries, grapes, and other dark red or blueberries deserve special mention, for they are rich sources of compounds that improve collagen metabolism, reduce joint inflammation, and relieve the symptoms of gout. The famous botanist Linnaeus reportedly cured his gout by eating large quantities of strawberries morning and night, which led him to call them "a blessing of the gods." More recently, a gout "strawberry cure" of eating nothing but strawberries for several days was made popular by the French herbalist Maurice Messegue. Many holistic physicians prescribe at least ½ cup of cherries daily for their arthritis patients, in keeping with that fruit's well-established reputation as a cure. When fresh fruit is not in season, gout patients report relief from eating canned and even candied cherries, but for best results, focus on fresh, frozen, or dried fruit.

The same herbs recommended for arthritis bring temporary relief from the symptoms of gout.

FIBROMYALGIA

Also known as fibrositis, fibromyalgia is a form of arthritis that most often strikes women between the ages of twenty and fifty, leaving them with sharp, stabbing aches and pains in the neck, knees, inner elbows, upper thigh, lower back, and hip areas, usually with accompanying sleep disturbances, ongoing fatigue, and occasionally serious depression. Some researchers believe that fibromyalgia victims share an underlying genetic susceptibility that lies dormant until triggered by a viral or bacterial infection, emotional trauma, or accident. In most cases, according to these experts, patients can trace their first symptoms to a specific event. Once established, the condition is often chronic, though the severity of symptoms may increase and decrease periodically.

According to rheumatologists, fibromyalgia is often misdiagnosed as chronic fatigue syndrome, for its victims are often exhausted, but fibromyalgia does not involve swollen lymph nodes or low-grade fever. The American College of Rheumatology publishes guidelines for physicians in which fibrositis/fibromyalgia is diagnosed if the patient has pain in eleven or more of the eighteen "tender points" mapped for this condition.

Food sensitivities play a role in fibromyalgia, just as they do in every other form of arthritis and rheumatism. Some people with no previous symptoms of arthritis or fibromyalgia experience severe muscle pain in the illness's key tender points after eating large amounts of animal protein, foods associated with allergic reactions such as shrimp, peanuts, or strawberries, or a combination of foods that for some reason triggers a response. Sugar, synthetic vitamins, and insufficient levels of essential fatty acids may also contribute to the disease.

Systemic oral enzyme therapy (see pages 91 to 92) helps treat and prevent fibromyalgia. Malic acid has been shown to help those with fibromyalgia, especially in combination with magnesium. Andrew Weil, M.D., recommends taking 200 to 250 milligrams of the amino acid L-carnitine twice daily on an empty stomach in addition to 300 to 600 milligrams of magnesium, and 1,200 to 2,400 milligrams of malic acid per day.

Dr. Weil also notes that the homeopathic remedy *Rhus tox*, derived from minute amounts of poison ivy, was found in one study to significantly reduce pain in fibromyalgia patients. For best results, consult an experienced homeopath to determine the correct remedy strength and dosage.

All of the herbs recommended for arthritis help relieve the pain of fibromyalgia.

CHAPTER TEN

Breathing Freely

THE WORD "ALLERGY" DID NOT exist in Shakespeare's time or even a hundred years ago. It's a modern term for a modern illness—or, more accurately, an assortment of illnesses. Allergy is a catchall word for a variety of reactions made by the body when it detects something foreign. The offending substances may be foods, animal dander, house dust, pollens, mold, smoke, air pollution, medicines, or chemicals. The ability of the immune system to identify individual substances and react to them is crucial, but overreaction creates uncomfortable symptoms such as sneezing, sinus congestion, itching or watery eyes, headaches, indigestion, skin rashes, hives, and other symptoms.

At any time of year, it can be hard to tell the difference between allergies and cold symptoms. Either can produce sneezes, a runny nose, nasal congestion, an itchy throat, and an irritated cough. If a "cold" lasts for several weeks, and if your symptoms seem more severe in certain locations (less intense outdoors in winter, for example, and worse in certain rooms or buildings), it's probably an allergic reaction or hay fever.

The link between diet and allergies is important, and anyone hoping to relieve hay fever symptoms and allergic reactions to dust mites, pet dander, and other common irritants will do well to explore food sensitivities. A mild reaction to pets combined with a mild reaction to tree pollen can become a major allergy attack when the immune system is further challenged by a meal containing wheat, dairy products, or other foods to which the person is sensitive.

THE HAY FEVER HONEY CURE

Honey contains pollen, and some hay fever sufferers swear by honey from local bees. They eat comb-honey or raw, unheated, unrefined, unfiltered honey from nearby hives, in three-day cycles for several weeks before hay fever season. This exposure acts like a vaccination and makes local pollens less irritating.

Bee pollen is a popular food supplement, but it can be dangerous to those who have hay fever. Some seriously adverse reactions have been reported among people with severe allergies who have taken bee pollen, probably because the typical dose is far more concentrated than what one would ingest in a spoonful of honey.

A more cautious approach is to start with a single grain of local bee pollen per day, three to four months before hay fever season, and slowly increase the dosage, adding one grain every three days. Discontinue if you experience any adverse symptoms, such as sinus congestion, throat irritation, fatigue, headaches, nausea, abdominal pain, diarrhea, itchy skin, or memory problems, all of which may occur when someone allergic to pollen takes bee pollen capsules daily for several weeks. The physician who reported these symptoms noted that bee pollen capsules, despite manufacturer's claims, do not contain only pollen from plants that are pollinated by bees but also allergenic airborne pollens such as ragweed.

A similar strategy is used by people who take ragweed tincture in the spring and early summer, before ragweed flowers. In-

spired when I read that Edgar Cayce had recommended ragweed tincture as a liver tonic and treatment for hay fever, I gathered blossoms from the inconspicuous common ragweed
(*Artemisia artemisifolia*) and the tree-tall great or giant ragweed
(*A. trifida*), covered the pollen-rich flowers with vodka, and
made my own tincture. The following spring I began taking
half a dropperful daily. All through ragweed season, which lasts
to the end of October, I continued the ragweed experiment and
seldom sneezed, even when pollen counts hit record highs.

HERBAL THERAPIES

Ma huang, also called Chinese ephedra, is the active ingredient
in most herbal allergy products. It clears bronchial passageways,
dries sinuses, helps relieve sneezing, and makes breathing easier.
It also speeds the pulse, raises blood pressure, makes it difficult to
relax, and feels like caffeine. The more you take, the more dramatic these side effects, so start with a small amount, don't take
Ma huang in the evening (it may keep you awake) and, if brewing a tea with this herb, make a weak infusion to start. For more
about Ma huang/ephedra, see page 134.

Nettle may sting when you touch it, but it compensates by
being one of the most important all-purpose tonic herbs. When
researchers tested hay fever patients with capsules containing
freeze-dried nettle, most improved dramatically within a week.
Although they weren't tested in double-blind, placebo-controlled
clinical trials, other nettle preparations, including tea, tincture, capsules, and extracts, have helped many hay fever victims stop sneezing. Nettle tea and fresh nettle juice are used in Europe for many
conditions, including respiratory problems.

Echinacea and goldenseal are a favorite combination for hay fever; in fact, some herbalists consider goldenseal the most effective botanical treatment for acute sinus infections because it fights bacteria and viruses while soothing mucous membranes. Both herbs support the immune system. Teas and tinctures made with red clover, sage, burdock root, or licorice root are often recommended for hay fever prevention and treatment, and all have much to recommend them.

The late Gail Ulrich, herbalist and director of the Blazing Star Herbal School, recommended an infusion of dried mullein leaf (2 tablespoons or 1 ounce by volume of the dried herb per quart of boiling water) steeped two to four hours and given in ½ cup doses four times daily for six weeks to eliminate allergies to pet dander and relieve other allergy symptoms.

Rosemary Gladstar has an unusual recipe for garlic-ginger syrup that helps prevent allergies and hay fevers. See page 223 for the recipe.

Saltwater solutions help clear nasal passages and relieve sinus congestion (see page 236).

A simple way to break the hay fever cycle without drugs is to go on a week-long cleansing juice fast, drinking only water and freshly prepared raw fruit and vegetable juices and eating no solid food at all. If you're like most hay fever sufferers, symptoms will diminish or disappear, suggesting a link to food sensitivities.

HOUSEPLANTS TO THE RESCUE

One effective air filter you don't have to send away for is the houseplant. When the National Aeronautics and Space Administration (NASA) discovered in 1973 that Skylab's tightly sealed air contained over a hundred toxic chemicals, the agency began a search for solutions. Learning that Russian scientists were experimenting with live plants as air purifiers, NASA hired research scientists to explore that possibility. The researchers found that all houseplants share the ability to purify air by pulling contaminants into their leaves. The toxins migrate to the roots and into the soil, where they decompose.

Trichlorethylene, formaldehyde, and benzene, three common pollutants, were treated in sealed growth chambers by common plants such as the peace lily, lady palm, and corn plant, any one of which could clean the air in a small (10 foot by 10 foot) room. As the study discovered, the more houseplants in a home or office, the more pure the air becomes. Other research has shown that the popular spider plant consumes tobacco smoke and that philodendrons and aloe vera are effective air purifiers.

To help your plant collection improve the quality of indoor air, place a layer of activated carbon at the bottom of each pot before adding soil; place a drop or two of grapefruit seed extract or tea tree oil or a tablespoon of topical hydrogen peroxide in drainage dishes every week before watering to prevent the growth of mold and bacteria in standing water; keep air circulating around plants with a low-speed fan; position plants at different heights; use a variety of plants; position shade-loving plants in areas that receive little or no natural light, and place sun-loving plants near windows; use at least one plant (two is better) for every 100 square feet of floor space in rooms of average height; and increase the number of plants for rooms with high ceilings, in areas in which cigarettes are smoked, or in homes near busy highways. Where necessary, supplement natural light with plant lights. Feed and water your green friends and they will repay you handsomely.

While mold can be a problem in greenhouses and other

humid, plant-filled spaces, carefully tended houseplants don't have to promote the growth of mold. The most common source of this problem is over-watered plants that stand on carpeting. Any carpet that becomes saturated and prevented from drying out will develop a serious mold and mildew infestation. Anyone concerned about potential pathogens in potting soil can prevent its contact with the air by spreading several inches of aquarium gravel over the top of the soil, or spraying the surface with a dilute solution of grapefruit seed extract and water. For a wealth of information on indoor gardening, see your local library, and visit nurseries and plant stores.

PETS AND THEIR DANDER

Dogs, cats, and other animals generate dander, a dandrufflike substance that consists of skin particles and, in animals that groom themselves, dried saliva. Animal dander is blamed for allergic reactions in adults and children, a worsening of asthma, and related respiratory problems.

Even pet-free homes contain dander. Feather pillows, down comforters, and some silk-filled comforters contain dander that commercial cleaning does not remove. Genuine oriental rugs and antique furniture stuffed with animal hair are sources of goat, sheep, or camel dander. Wool from underdeveloped countries is a common source of sheep dander, unlike domestic wool that is processed to be dander-free. Angora sweaters and inexpensive rabbit "fun furs" are a source of dander that can't be washed away because of the fibers' fragility. Pet birds are a serious source of allergens, not because their feathers are allergenic but because they, too, harbor dander. Even lawns and gardens can be a seasonal source of cattle dander, for it appears in large amounts in cow manure, a popular fertilizer.

Because animal dander triggers so many adverse reactions, allergists often recommend that pets be given away. In twenty years of doctor appointments for the treatment of hay fever and asthma, I was usually told on the first office visit to get rid of my cats. Like many pet lovers who receive this prescription, I refused. None of my dozen doctors offered alternative solutions; all announced in authoritative voices that there was no way to remove the problem without removing the pets, and all but one expressed annoyance and irritation at patients who refused to cooperate.

But for every study that links pet dander to respiratory problems, others show that pet owners live longer, have happier lives, have lower stress levels, and enjoy more meaningful relationships than those who don't share their lives with pets. Nursing homes with resident pets have lower death rates, lower infection rates, and lower staff turnover rates than those without. A study of recovering heart attack victims showed that the most significant difference between those who died within one year and those who survived was dog ownership. For many Americans, pets are members of the family. Getting rid of them, even on a doctor's orders, is as traumatic as losing a relative.

Pet dander in carpeted homes is more of a problem than in homes with bare floors, although any rug or fabric can harbor dander. The source of the problem isn't hair that the animals shed but proteins in their saliva and flakes of skin. Young kittens and puppies seldom trigger allergic reactions; they have no old skin to shed and therefore no dander. It isn't until the age of three or four months, or even later, that pets begin to produce the allergen. This explains how someone can develop a sudden allergy to a pet that was for months a comfortable roommate.

Cleaning equipment that sprays hot water and vacuums it up removes dander from rugs and carpets more efficiently than plain vacuuming. Dogs and cats that eat a natural, raw-meat diet produce far less dander than animals fed commercial pet food. For information on home-prepared diets, see my books *The Encyclopedia of Natural Pet Care* and *Natural Remedies for Dogs and Cats*. Rinsing a pet once a week removes dander before it causes problems. Pet stores offer allergy grooming solutions that can be applied with a damp cloth or sprayed onto dogs, cats, and birds, but plain water or herbal tea works well, too. Don't use soap; it's harsh, strips away protective oils, and is difficult to rinse out. The secret to success in using any pet allergy product is making sure the product reaches your pet's skin.

My husband's red tabby, Pumpkin, was famous for his love of water. Every week I filled a spray bottle with lukewarm chamomile tea (recommended for blondes and redheads—human, canine, and feline), sat on the floor, spread towels on my lap, and soaked him to the skin while he purred and kneaded. After a vigorous drying off, he would lie in the sun until his fur was once again gorgeous, fluffy, sweet smelling, and nonallergenic.

Of course, in some cases, radical measures are necessary. Some families have to find new homes for their pets when other measures fail to prevent life-threatening asthma attacks. The strategies described here don't work for everyone, but what many pet owners don't realize is that alternatives exist at all. I believe they're worth trying before dogs and cats are banished from any caring home.

ASTHMA

A full-blown asthma attack is a nightmare: you can't catch your breath. Add coughing, rattly wheezing, a choking sensation, and the lightheaded feeling that accompanies a lack of oxygen, and you get the idea. Asthma is worse than inconvenient; it can be fatal. In the United States, asthma has become an epidemic, especially among children. Orthodox physicians treat it with steroids, antihistamines, bronchiole dilators, and other drugs, all of which have adverse side effects and none of which address asthma's cause.

"Extrinsic" or "atopic" asthma is related to allergies and brings a characteristic increase in the blood serum immunoglobulin IgE. "Intrinsic" asthma does not involve allergies; it is triggered by chemicals, exposure to cold air or water, active physical exercise, infection, or emotional upset. No matter what conditions trigger an asthma attack, naturopathic physicians believe that asthma's underlying causes are food sensitivities and exposure to food additives and other chemicals that overburden the immune system and cause it to malfunction. Diets that eliminate common allergens have been effective in treating asthmatic adults and children. Double-blind food challenges in children have shown sensitivities that result in immediate symptoms are most likely to involve eggs, fish, shellfish, nuts, and peanuts, while those that result in the delayed onset of symptoms are most likely to involve milk, chocolate, wheat, citrus fruits, and food coloring. Of course, every person is different, and the best way to tell what foods may be triggering your or your child's symptoms is to keep a food diary, experiment with food groups and rotation diets, or see a health care professional who specializes in nutrition.

In someone whose production of hydrochloric acid is insufficient for complete digestion, discovering food allergies is only part of the problem, for unless the low stomach acid is corrected, new food sensitivities will develop as new foods replace old ones. According to Jonathan Wright, M.D., one of the diseases associated with low stomach acid is childhood asthma. This deficiency is easy to diagnose and the cure is inexpensive (see page 87).

In 1993, *The American Journal of Epidemiology* reported on a study that compared 457 asthmatic children ages three to four with 457 control subjects. Independent risk factors for asthma included heavy smoking by the mother and the use of a humidifier in the child's room. Less important but still significant were the presence of other smokers in the home, a history of pneumonia, the absence of breast-feeding, and a family history of asthma. Other studies have shown that smoke from a fireplace or wood stove can aggravate asthma, as can a host of common household cleansers, paints, paint thinners, perfumes, and some types of incense.

Mold and Mildew

The problem with humidifiers, which are supposed to help relieve respiratory congestion, is that they are breeding grounds for molds, bacteria, and other germs. To prevent these problems, add liquid grapefruit seed extract or a solution of tea tree oil (see page 163) to your humidifier's water reservoir.

A 1984 study published in *The New England Journal of Medicine* found that almost one out of every five people with asthma or allergies experienced symptoms from their car air conditioner. The culprit was mold, which affected nearly all the cars tested. This condition, most prevalent in warm, humid climates, usually generates an unpleasant odor. In response, auto makers have developed an air-conditioning odor treatment that eliminates and prevents the growth of molds, yeast, bacteria, and viruses. Check with dealers or service centers for solutions to the car air-conditioning problem.

Cockroaches and Dust Mites

One overlooked producer of household allergens is the cockroach. An estimated 20 to 30 percent of hospital admissions relating to asthma and indoor allergies in urban areas may be caused by cockroach sensitization. Many insecticides are guaranteed to kill cockroaches, but they are not recommended for use around asthma patients or anyone with a compromised immune system. Immaculate housekeeping and the storage of food in sealed plastic or glass containers makes any kitchen unattractive to insects. The essential oils of thyme, lemongrass, lavender, peppermint, tea tree, and citronella have insect-repelling properties. They can be dabbed on cupboard walls or mixed with water and applied with a damp sponge to help repel cockroaches.

A similar source of irritation is the dust mite, which has been shown to worsen symptoms in asthma patients as well as allergy sufferers.

To reduce exposure to dust mites, some experts recommend putting sheets, pillows, and pillowcases in a hot dryer twice a week for ten minutes; keeping stuffed animals, shaggy rugs, quilts, and dolls out of the bedroom; having pets sleep away from the bedroom; and frequently rinsing one's face in hot, salted water.

Another treatment for dust mites is tea tree oil. A dilute solution (0.8 percent tea tree oil) can be made by combining ½ tablespoon tea tree oil with 2 tablespoons vodka or other alcohol to make it water-dispersible and adding 1 quart of water. Exposure to a 0.8 percent solution of tea tree oil kills 100 percent of treated dust mites within thirty minutes. Where rinsing or sponging is inconvenient, the solution can be sprayed. It can be applied to carpets through any rug shampoo appliance.

Food Additives

Medical research has linked asthma to a variety of food additives, especially sulfites and monosodium glutamate (MSG). Sulfites have been known to cause asthma, anaphylaxis, abdominal pain, hives, seizures, and in some cases death. The flavor enhancer MSG is blamed for Chinese restaurant syndrome and the immediate or late triggering of asthma. The orange food coloring tartrazine, found in jams, jellies, candies, cakes, some brands of butter, and some tablets, can cause both hives and asthma.

Restaurants used to use sulfites to keep cut vegetables from changing color, but in response to the growing demand for sulfite-free food, most have discontinued this practice. Sulfite test strips are available from most pharmacies, making it easy to check unfamiliar foods for these additives. Some popular beverages targeted at children contain colored water, sugar, flavoring, and sulfites. Always check product labels.

A Japanese physician at the National Children's Hospital in Tokyo has discovered that cold water may cure some asthmas. As David Williams, M.D., reported in the May 1994 edition of his newsletter *Alternatives*, Dr. Toshio Katsunuma conducted a study of twenty-five asthmatic children ages four to twenty. Each child was given a cold shower every day, in which twenty buckets of 59-degree Fahrenheit water were poured over the child for one minute. Twenty other patients received a warmer shower, in which the water was 86 degrees Fahrenheit. There was no change in the warm water group, but all of the cold water group required less asthma medication, and some were able to discontinue medication altogether. None of the cold water treatments triggered an asthma attack. Dr. Williams remarked, "I doubt there's a kid anywhere who wouldn't rather take a one-minute cold shower every morning than put up with the side effects and social stigma of asthma medication and inhalers."

Because exposure to cold water can trigger intrinsic asthma attacks, this approach is the opposite of what most American physicians recommend. But a cold-water shower, approached cautiously and in the absence of any history of asthma triggered by exposure to cold air or water, is a simple experiment.

Herbs for Asthma

Herbs have a vital place in asthma therapy. The most frequently prescribed include echinacea, horsetail, juniper berries, licorice root, mullein, and Ma huang. Lobelia tincture may be helpful during asthma attacks, as it relaxes bronchial muscles. Ginkgo, which contains the active ingredient ginkgolide B, has shown good results in many studies.

According to the herbalist Christopher Hobbes, teas or extracts of the expectorant herbs grindelia and yerba santa are best for asthma accompanied by a heavy white sputum, while the moisturizing herbs coltsfoot, marshmallow root, mullein, and licorice are better for asthma accompanied by dry coughs.

Wheat grass juice and powders are often used to help patients with respiratory disorders, and now an Australian extract of rye grass (see Oralmat in the Resources section) is being used to treat asthma, allergies, and other conditions.

Mullein, a common roadside plant, is another specific for asthma. New York herbalist Robin Bennett has seen asthma attacks interrupted by lighting dry mullein leaves, blowing the flame out, and inhaling the smoke. Someone assisting can hold a fireproof container (such as an ashtray) of smoking leaves within a few inches of the person's face until normal breathing resumes, which usually takes place in less than sixty seconds. This simple procedure has been effective in adults and children, even during serious attacks. "One of my first experiences as an apprentice herbalist with Susun Weed," Bennett told me, "was to smoke a mullein cigarette with her so that I could experience for myself the feeling of my bronchioles dilating in response to the soothing smoke. This is another traditional way of using mullein for asthma."

Bennett's students report that drinking a strong, mullein leaf infusion daily helps reduce the frequency and severity of asthma attacks. Some have successfully weaned themselves off all asthma medication, such as one runner who found herself able to complete her run without having to stop and use her inhaler. In addition, Bennett suggests the use of positive affirmations, such as "I deserve to breathe freely," as reminders that deep, comfortable, healthy breathing is each person's right. "Self-worth is often an issue," she explained. "Whatever a person can do to increase his or her self-esteem is a powerful treatment for asthma."

My teacher, Rosemary Gladstar, shares with all her students a recipe that helps prevent and treat asthma, hay fever, bronchial inflammation, coughs, and colds. Many years ago in California, Hari Das Baba led a series of small retreats in the Occidental Hills. This wise man had not spoken a word for years, but in answer to his students' questions he wrote brilliant answers on a chalkboard.

For days Gladstar pondered all the cosmic questions in her mind, trying to decide which one to ask. Finally her turn arrived. With reverence and solemn eagerness, she asked, "What is the best recipe you know of for asthma and hay fever?" The recipe he shared makes a remarkable garlic-ginger syrup. "Make at least one or two quarts," says Gladstar. "You'll use it all!"

Garlic-Ginger Syrup

Juice equal parts fresh gingerroot and fresh garlic in a juicer. Combine the juices in a saucepan and sweeten with just enough honey to thicken, usually ¼ to ½ cup honey per cup of juice. Warm the mixture just enough to mix in the honey but do not overheat. Remove from the stove and add enough cayenne pepper to make it taste hot, sweet, spicy, and pungent.

Pour the mixture into a glass jar, wrap it in a blanket or large towel, and cover with a paper bag. Find an appropriate place in or near your garden, dig a hole, bury the jar, and leave it in the ground for seventeen days. At the end of this time, it is ready to use. Suggested dosage: 1 teaspoon three times daily, as needed.

When I first made the syrup, I seasoned it with Tabasco sauce and left it in the ground for four months, a variation on the guru's recipe. Fermentation and the passage of time produced a stunning blend of flavors. My husband used it to season his stir-fried rice. When a friend had a cold that wouldn't go away, complete with a hacking cough that left his throat raw, we gave him an 8-ounce bottle. Taking a swig every half hour, he finished the bottle in one night. By morning, his cold had disappeared without a trace. Even his sore throat felt fine. Warning: the garlic odor is overwhelming, but when you really want to feel better, that doesn't matter.

If you don't have four months or even seventeen days to spare, you can use the same ingredients in other ways. Ginger and cayenne are warming, stimulant herbs, and garlic is an all-purpose infection fighter. They work well in combination with other herbs and can be added to any treatment involving capsules, tinctures, and/or teas.

Aromatherapy

Although many essential oils are described as treatments for asthma, Dr. Kurt Schnaubelt writes in *Advanced Aromatherapy* that essential oils do not offer a miracle cure for the disease. "Nonetheless," he says, "in many cases aromatherapy does relieve symptoms." Success depends, he believes, on how far the illness has progressed with conventional treatment. Asthma patients who have experienced breathing problems but are not yet dependent on prescription medication are most likely to benefit from the therapy he describes.

If the patient is unfamiliar with essential oils, Schnaubelt suggests a gradual reconditioning of her appreciation of fragrance. To someone exclusively accustomed to synthetic aromas, the purity and potency of genuine essential oils may seem overwhelming or unattractive. They take getting used to. To assist the transition, he recommends gentle massages with diluted essential oils that have widely accepted fragrances and good spasmolytic properties, such as lavender and mandarin, in a vegetable-oil base. Essential oils that harmonize well with lavender and mandarin are Roman chamomile, spikenard, and clary sage. "Experience has shown that asthma patients who react positively to these oils will soon begin to develop a positive attitude toward aromatherapy," he explains.

The second phase introduces stronger oils that are more specifically geared to the asthma condition, such as *Eucalyptus radiata* or *Ravensare aromatica*, both of which have expectorant and antiasthmatic effects. Instead of being diluted in a carrier oil, these are applied freely to wet skin during or after a shower. If the patient reacts positively to those measures, a third phase addresses his specific symptoms with essential oil blends that are inhaled, swallowed in gelatin capsules, or applied in a suppository base of cocoa butter.

In *Aromatherapy for Common Ailments*, British aromatherapist Shirley Price recommends sprinkling a few drops each of cajeput, atlas cedarwood, and eucalyptus essential oils on a tissue, and inhaling deeply three times with eyes closed before placing the tissue close to the chest. In an emergency, she says, place 1 drop of cajeput oil into your palm, cup both hands together, and cover the nose, inhaling deeply. She does not recommend inhaling essential oils over a bowl of hot water during an asthma attack because concentrated steam can cause choking.

In addition, a massage oil containing 3 drops atlas cedarwood, 2 drops peppermint, and 1 drop cajeput essential oil diluted in 4 teaspoons carrier oil can be applied to the chest, throat, and upper back.

BRONCHITIS

Bronchitis is defined as an acute (intense and sudden) or chronic (long standing) inflammation of the mucous lining of the bronchial tubes, the main airway to the lungs. Acute bronchitis often develops after an upper respiratory infection, such as a cold or the flu. The resulting cough is at first very dry but it becomes less painful and rasping as the lungs produce mucus, which lubricates the bronchi. In some cases, bronchitis may be followed by pneumonia. If a fever lasts for more than a few days, complications are likely.

Statistics show that smokers are more likely to die from chronic bronchitis than from lung cancer, so for smokers, the best strategy is to quit.

Foods such as wheat (especially white flour), refined carbohydrates, sugar, and dairy products often exacerbate chronic bronchitis. By experimenting with diet, eliminating processed foods, dairy products, and wheat while increasing the consumption of raw foods, many have reduced or eliminated their bronchitis symptoms. Garlic is often recommended as a food supplement, along with vitamins, minerals, and "green" foods such as wheat grass, barley grass, spirulina, and chlorella.

Expectorant herbs are important for relief of the exhausting cough that comes with bronchitis, but the type of herb depends on the type of cough. For relief from a dry, hacking, irritating cough, use a relaxing expectorant such as coltsfoot or lobelia; for a wet cough, use a stimulating expectorant like horehound or elecampane.

The famous Austrian herbalist Maria Treben recommended breathing steam from coltsfoot flowers and leaves to relieve bronchitis. Pour boiling water over fresh or dried coltsfoot, then drape a towel over your head and the bowl to retain the resulting steam.

Steam inhalations using coltsfoot or other herbs are soothing in all stages of bronchitis. Add 1 teaspoon each of chamomile blossoms, thyme, and marjoram to 2 cups boiling water, or add any of the following essential oils to a bowl of steaming water: bergamot, eucalyptus, fir, lavender, peppermint, sage, sandalwood, tea tree oil, thyme, or white pine. Peppermint oil may be most effective in the early stages of bronchitis.

In *An Elder's Herbal*, David Hoffmann recommends osha, a plant native to the American Southwest, as "an excellent specific in cases of tracheobronchitis." Osha root, which has a sharp and pungent taste, can be chewed for relief from coughs and sore throats. For all bronchitis symptoms, he recommends a tea made of equal parts mullein, coltsfoot, marshmallow, and aniseed; pour 1 cup boiling water over 2 cups dried herbs and let stand, covered, for ten minutes. Drink several cups daily. For bronchitis accompanied by a wet cough, Hoffmann suggests 1 tablespoon of an expectorant tincture made of equal parts elecampane, horehound, coltsfoot, goldenseal, and echinacea, taken three times daily.

As the patient recovers from bronchitis, coltsfoot, horehound, and mullein are especially useful given as teas or tinctures several times daily.

The same essential oils used for asthma are recommended for bronchitis.

COLDS AND FLU

We associate viral diseases with winter or with a change of season, but you can catch a cold or the flu at any time. What's the difference? Both cause respiratory distress, fever, coughing, headaches, sore throat, aching muscles, and fatigue, but the flu (short for influenza) is usually more severe, faster developing, and involves more of the body. Vomiting and diarrhea are common flu symptoms.

If you're serious about staying well, it makes sense to improve your diet, reduce the stress in your life, and avoid the foods, drugs, and pollutants that suppress immunity. These include sugar, junk food, and cigarettes, as well as chemicals, pesticides, and air pollutants.

Left alone, most colds go away by themselves within a week, but with the help of certain herbs, your symptoms can disappear much faster.

Mention colds and flu to most herbalists and they will recommend echinacea. The purple cone flower, *Echinacea purpurea*, and its narrow-leaved relative, *E. angustifolia*, have been shown to increase T-cell activity and related immune system activity. When taken in the early stages of illness, echinacea wards off viral infections and is very effective when taken frequently, in large doses, for brief periods.

Echinacea is often combined with goldenseal or Oregon grape root, both of which contain berberine, a strong antibiotic substance. Goldenseal enhances immune function by stimulating circulation to the spleen and toning the lymph system. Echinacea and goldenseal work well with licorice root, an herb that supports the immune system through its effect on the adrenal glands. Tinctures containing these combinations are widely sold, or make your own for even better results. See the instructions for making effective tinctures on pages 147 to 148.

I learned to appreciate echinacea and goldenseal when a wet blizzard soaked me to the skin. My teeth chattered so loudly my husband said they sounded like castanets. My bones felt frozen, and I sneezed and coughed all over everything. Most unpleasant! Beginning that afternoon, I took ¼ teaspoon of a combined echinacea and goldenseal tincture every half hour plus a gram of food-source vitamin C every hour until I fell asleep at midnight. The next morning, not only had every trace of illness disappeared but I felt better than I had in months. This strategy works best if used on the first day of cold symptoms.

Astragalus root is an increasingly popular Chinese herb used to flavor soups and rice dishes. Chinese research has shown it to increase activity of the immune system, and it's easy to add a piece to whatever you're cooking to boost winter immunity.

Chicken soup has a long medicinal history, dating back to the twelfth-century physician Moses Maimonides, who is said to have prescribed it for the Muslim Sultan Saladin. Chicken contains cysteine, an amino acid that closely resembles acetylcysteine, which doctors prescribe for respiratory infections. In 1978, Marvin Sackner, M.D., a pulmonary specialist at Mount Sinai Medical School in Florida, conducted a now-famous "chicken soup" study. Fifteen healthy men and women sipped hot chicken soup, hot water, or cold water out of covered and uncovered containers, after which their mucus and airflow rates were measured. Chicken soup and its vapors relieved congestion better than either the hot or cold water.

Irwin Ziment, M.D., a professor of medicine at the University of California, Los Angeles and an authority on traditional remedies, prescribes spicy foods for colds, sinusitis, asthma, hay fever, emphysema, and chronic bronchitis because peppers and other spices perform as well as many over-the-counter drugs, but without their adverse side effects. Dr. Ziment calls spicy chicken soup "the best cold remedy there is," especially when flavored with garlic, onion, pepper, curry, or chili peppers. To prevent colds and flu, he prescribes a bowl of spicy chicken soup daily. Vegetarians can substitute miso, a Japanese fermented soybean paste, for chicken in a similarly spicy broth.

Andrew Weil, M.D., prefers natural remedies to pharmaceuticals and his favorite cold cure is garlic. "Eat several cloves of raw garlic at the first onset of symptoms," he recommends. "Cut it in chunks and swallow them whole like pills. If it gives you flatulence, eat less." Dr. Weil prescribes one or two cloves of garlic to anyone who suffers from chronic or recurrent infections or low resistance to infection.

For Rosemary Gladstar's garlic-ginger syrup, which helps cure colds and flu, see page 223. To treat accompanying sinus congestion, see the instructions for nasal rinsing on pages 233 and 234.

To treat chest congestion, combine congestion-clearing essential oils with a carrier oil such as olive or almond oil to make a soothing chest balm. Peppermint, eucalyptus, and tea tree oils work well for this purpose.

COUGHS

Coughing is a reflex response to anything that interferes with the passage of air to the lungs. In most cases, the cause is mucus secreted by membranes lining the respiratory tract.

The breathless cough of an asthma attack can be treated with mullein, including the smoke of burning mullein leaf (see page 222). When anxiety contributes to asthma, nervines like oatstraw, chamomile, and lobelia help prevent spasms and coughing.

As noted in the section describing bronchitis, dry, hacking, irritating coughs respond well to relaxing expectorants like lobelia and coltsfoot, while wet coughs need more stimulating expectorants such as horehound and elecampane.

When an illness such as a cold or the flu causes coughing, the use of cough-suppressing herbs interferes with the body's cleansing mechanisms, for coughing helps the body rid itself of waste products. In that case, expectorant herbs such as horehound and coltsfoot are effective, because they make coughing more productive. Infection-fighting herbs such as echinacea and the culinary herbs sage and thyme are also helpful, for they help remove the cause of the illness.

Whenever coughing produces blood or does not respond to treatment and lasts more than a week, it should be checked by a medical professional.

Herbalist Gail Ulrich used the following cough syrup for colds, flu, and other respiratory problems. First, blend equal parts wild cherry bark, licorice root, and burdock root, then add a smaller amount (¼ to ½ part) osha root. In a 1-quart jar place 2 tablespoons of this herbal blend, cover with boiling water, close the jar, and let the tea steep for at least four hours or overnight. Next, blend equal parts of dried mullein leaf, sage, coltsfoot, and comfrey leaf, then add a small amount (¼ part) peppermint and, for adults, an equal amount of horehound. Place 2 tablespoons of this tea in a 1-quart mason jar, add boiling water, close the lid, and let the tea stand for two hours.

Strain and combine these two teas in a large saucepan, and simmer uncovered until the tea is reduced to one-half or, for a stronger syrup, one-quarter of its volume. For every cup of tea add 3 to 4 tablespoons honey or a combination of 2 tablespoons honey and 2 tablespoons black cherry concentrate. Add a splash of brandy as a preservative and use as needed to soothe a sore throat.

EMPHYSEMA

Now known officially as chronic obstructive pulmonary disease or COPD, emphysema often accompanies chronic bronchitis. It is caused by a lack of elasticity in the lungs, usually due to constant coughing. When the lungs cannot expand and contract with ease, it is difficult to breathe. Emphysema often brings a distinctive deep wheezing that interrupts conversation and physical movement. It is so debilitating that it ranks third among the diseases for which Social Security gives disability benefits. Patients often have a history of heavy smoking or live in areas of high air pollution.

The herbal treatments for emphysema are similar to those for asthma, with an added emphasis on nutritional support for the immune system. See the suggestions for asthma therapy. Some physicians prescribe a low-carbohydrate diet because sweets, simple carbohydrates, and sugar tend to worsen emphysema symptoms.

Vitamins C and E, magnesium, and bioflavonoids are important supplements for those with emphysema and so are omega-3 fish oils. In 1994, *The New England Journal of Medicine* reported on a study of nearly nine thousand smokers and former smokers that showed the more fish they ate, the less chance they had of developing emphysema.

Several studies have shown that emphysema patients do well when oxygen is administered continuously, especially at night. Two trials in the 1980s showed a 50 percent improvement in the rate of death when people with COPD received continuous oxygen therapy. Now hyperbaric oxygen therapy, which saturates the system with oxygen under pressure, is beginning to be used for this disease.

The relaxing expectorant herbs lobelia and coltsfoot can be helpful in treating emphysema, as can elecampane. A tea made of equal parts coltsfoot, lobelia, and the soothing demulcent herbs mullein and Irish moss may help reduce coughing and shortness of breath. Add an equal amount of licorice root if high blood pressure and fluid retention are not a problem. Use 1 to 2 teaspoons tea per cup of boiling water; brew 4 cups at a time in a quart jar for convenience, reheat as desired, and sip throughout the day.

SINUS CONGESTION

A symptom of hay fever allergies and colds or flu, sinus congestion makes breathing difficult. Chronic sinusitis sometimes follows these illnesses, causing a dull ache around the eyes and face. Swimming in the ocean is one way to relieve congestion; another is to create the same effect while standing over the bathroom sink. Hand-held ceramic containers with long spouts have become popular for this purpose (see the Neti Pot in the Resources). Similar designs are available in some health food stores and catalogs. If you can't find a Neti Pot, ask your pharmacist for a nasal douche apparatus or simply hold saltwater in your hand and sniff it up one nostril while you hold the other closed. The more saltwater that irrigates sinus passages, the greater relief. Use enough so the water drains out through your mouth, washing away debris as it does.

To disinfect as you rinse, use warm sage or thyme tea instead of plain water and add a pinch of salt, or do as Dr. Penoel recommends and mix 8 tablespoons unrefined sea salt in a small jar with 3 milliliters (approximately 36 drops) tea tree oil and 1 milliliter (12 drops) verbenone-type or cineole-type rosemary. Stir well with a wooden chopstick. Seal the jar when not in use to preserve the essential oils.

Add 1 to 2 teaspoons of the aromatic salt to about 2 cups warm water, stir well, and use this solution to irrigate the sinuses. Dr. Penoel's preferred method of application is with a HydroFloss irrigator, an electric appliance for tooth and gum care, but any procedure that rinses the sinuses will work.

Facial steam baths help clear sinus passages to allow free breathing. This therapy can be as simple as holding your head over a steaming bowl of chicken soup when you have a cold. If you have a facial sauna, sold in beauty supply shops and some pharmacies, plug it in and inhale. If desired, add a drop of tea tree, eucalyptus, sage, ginger, or rosemary essential oil, all of which are decongestants. Alternatively, pour boiling water into a bowl to which you have added a few drops of essential oil. Make a tent of a large towel to cover your head and the bowl, then breathe the medicated steam for several minutes. Keep your head well above the bowl to prevent scalding, and come out for air as necessary.

The herbs Ma huang and goldenseal are specifics for sinus problems. Astringent herbs such as goldenrod, eyebright, and elder flower contain tannins that help dry up excess mucus. Echinacea and garlic fight upper respiratory infections. And don't forget diet. A major cause of chronic sinusitis is food sensitivities. In addition to using herbs that help relieve symptoms, a new diet may eliminate the condition altogether.

SORE THROAT

The pain of a sore throat makes any illness worse. One traditional treatment is to gargle with saltwater or a strong herbal tea several times a day, spitting the gargle solution out without swallowing. Add a teaspoon of salt to a cup of water or warm tea for this purpose. If you can sing and gargle at the same time, the soothing liquid will contact more throat surface.

Licorice root tea soothes throat soreness and reduces pain. Simmer 1 tablespoon licorice root in 3 cups water, covered, for ten to fifteen minutes. Drink one cup three times daily unless you have high blood pressure or edema (fluid retention). Gargling with licorice root tea does not cause side effects.

Hot sage tea is a popular European remedy for sore throats. Steep 1 or 2 teaspoons dried sage leaves or 1 to 2 tablespoons fresh sage in 1 cup boiling water, covered, for ten minutes. Sip slowly or add salt and gargle.

Daniel Penoel considers tea tree oil one of the safest and most effective means of controlling and eliminating minor infections, especially cases of sore throat, pharyngitis, and other throat infections. The secret to success, he says, is immediate action. The moment you feel an unpleasant tickle at the back of the throat, place a drop on your tongue. If you don't have a bottle of tea tree oil with you, he warns, you won't have time to go out and buy one; it's important to be prepared and have one handy at all times.

Begin by placing a small amount on a fingertip and wipe the excess on the edge of the bottle opening. A trace amount is sufficient. Then place the finger on your tongue, diluting the oil with saliva. Bathe the entire mouth and throat as much as possible, then swallow. Repeat this application frequently, such as every minute for ten minutes. In addition, once or twice apply a drop to each side of the neck behind the ear and below the corner of the lower jaw.

Continue the treatment at less frequent intervals, such as

every five minutes for four to five repetitions, then every ten minutes, then every twenty minutes, and so on.

Alternatively, Dr. Penoel suggests diluting 4 drops of tea tree oil in 1 tablespoon honey; then take a pea-sized amount as described above. Unlike more toxic essential oils, tea tree oil can be mixed directly with honey and is safe for this type of internal use.

CHAPTER ELEVEN

Other Aches and Pains

HEADACHES

Headaches may be the world's most widely shared medical symptom. They can be caused by or accompany fevers, colds, allergy attacks, worry, stress, close work, eye strain, prescription drugs, certain odors, diseases such as hypertension, head or neck injuries, poor posture, pinched nerves, hormonal changes, menstruation, menopause, chemicals, and other environmental factors. In some cases, their cause remains a mystery. Headaches can be mild, or they can keep a victim bedridden for days. They may occur in cycles, disappear and never come back, recur in clusters, or never go away at all.

Migraines are the most painful and debilitating of headaches, often accompanied by flashing lights, nausea, blurred vision, and an unbearable feeling of fullness or pressure. These symptoms are caused by the narrowing of blood vessels resulting in reduced blood supply to parts of the brain, followed by expansion or dilation of the vessels.

Diet is the first line of defense in chasing headaches away. The prestigious British medical journal *The Lancet* reported in 1983 that the most common cause of migraine headache is food allergy. In carefully controlled studies, approximately 80 to 90 percent of migraine sufferers were shown to have food aller-gies. The most common offenders were milk and other dairy products, wheat, chocolate, eggs, and oranges. In a study of chil-dren with frequent migraines, 93 percent responded to an al-lergy elimination diet. Foods linked in other studies to all types of headaches include refined and processed foods (white flour, white sugar, white rice, commercial baked goods, etc.), coffee, tea, alcohol, red or white wine, soft drinks, grapes, plums, figs, bananas, dried fruits, lentils, kidney beans, nuts, onions, herring, chocolate, peanut butter, chicken livers, sour cream, yogurt, vinegar, pickled or fermented foods, foods containing mono-sodium glutamate (MSG), citrus fruit, processed meats, and ripened cheeses. West German research indicates that foods con-taining the amino acid tyramine, which can cause blood pressure to rise, may result in a dull headache. Foods rich in tyramine include bananas, cheese, sour cream, chicken, chocolate, citrus fruits, cold cuts, smoked fish, peanut butter, onions, pork, vine-gar, wine, and freshly baked yeast products.

When foods are the underlying cause of your headaches, keeping a food diary, following a four-day rotation diet, avoid-ing potentially troublesome foods for at least a week and then adding no more than one new food per day, or using the pulse test developed by Dr. A. Coca, can help reveal which foods are problematic. See chapter 3.

When it isn't possible to avoid a headache-triggering food, you may still be able to prevent that reaction. In their book, *Prescription for Nutritional Healing*, James and Phyllis Balch rec-ommend taking five charcoal tablets (available in health food stores) within an hour of the meal and an additional three tablets afterward. Charcoal tablets are not recommended for everyday use because they absorb nutrients as well as toxins, but they are safe for occasional preventive treatment.

Tension headaches sometimes respond to the simplest of therapies: deep breathing and lukewarm baths. Deep breathing exercises, such as stretching while inhaling and bending forward while exhaling, allowing the hands and arms to hang limply, help release tension and increase circulation and oxygen supply to the brain.

Physical exercise, such as brisk walking, helps some headaches disappear.

Slow, deep breathing helps relieve stress and increases blood circulation to the extremities. In early biofeedback experiments, people who learned how to warm their cold hands by relaxing and breathing slowly, discovered that their headaches went away as a result. When blood vessels dilate, blood flow to the extremities increases, reducing the blood vessel constriction that causes migraines.

Holding an ice pack or bag of frozen vegetables against the forehead while soaking the feet in hot water or a hot herbal tea may prevent a migraine headache; drinking three glasses of very cold water at the first sign of a headache, then resting with a cold compress in a dark quiet room without a pillow may prevent a tension headache; and inhaling pure oxygen from a tank kept in the bedroom may offset nighttime cluster headaches.

Both the consumption of caffeine and abrupt caffeine withdrawal can trigger headaches. If you drink coffee, tea, or colas containing caffeine, try to reduce your consumption gradually, not abruptly. Hangover headaches are caused by alcohol, which dilates and irritates blood vessels in the brain. Red wine, rum, port, brandy, and liqueurs cause the most serious discomfort. To help avoid a hangover headache, eat ripe fruit and vegetables or eat a little honey; drink alcohol slowly; drink additional water or tomato juice; and don't overindulge.

Because honey has been reported to have a balancing effect on the production of the brain chemical serotonin, some migraine and tension headache sufferers have experimented with a daily teaspoon of unpasteurized honey as well as a spoonful under the tongue at the first warning signs of a headache.

Low levels of the mineral magnesium may contribute to migraine and cluster headaches. Some experts recommend taking 200 milligrams of magnesium three times per day to help prevent these headaches, but smaller doses of food-source minerals are also effective. Taking a supplement that contains niacin (vitamin B_3) and niacinamide at the first sign of pain may keep blood vessels dilated, and prevent a migraine by reducing the initial constriction phase.

Herbs to the Rescue

Because headaches have plagued human beings since time began, there are thousands of herbal headache therapies. White willow bark (*Salix alba*) was the original aspirin, a natural source of salicin, though less concentrated and milder than its synthesized counterpart. White willow bark was used in ancient Egypt, Greece, and Assyria as well as by North American Indian tribes to treat headache, fever, arthritis, rheumatism, and other ailments. In his book *Natural Relief from Headaches, Insomnia & Stress*, David Hoffmann explains that willow bark is most useful in treating headaches that coincide with arthritis, sports injuries, and similar conditions that involve inflammation of the joints, muscles, and connective tissue, but that, like aspirin, it is less helpful in treating stress or tension heacaches. White willow bark is an ingredient in several herbal headache preparations, and it is sold separately as well.

Bentony, bergamot, basil, buck bean, calendula, cayenne, chamomile, elder flower, ground ivy, ginger, Jamaican dogwood, lady's slipper, lavender, lemon balm, marjoram, meadowsweet, nettle, parsley, passionflower, peppermint, rosemary, rue, sage, skullcap, speedwell, sweet marjoram, sweet woodruff, thyme, valerian, wood betony, wormwood, and yerba mate are just a few of the herbs recommended by herbalists around the world. Valerian and passionflower are especially helpful for tension headaches, as are blends of skullcap, valerian, and oat straw, or blends of hawthorn and skullcap. Ginger helps relieve the nausea associated with migraine headaches; the application of an ointment containing capsaicin (cayenne) to the inside of the nostrils several times a day may relieve cluster headaches; and the application of the same cayenne ointment to the skin may prevent migraines. Cayenne ointments are sold as over-the-counter arthritis pain relievers. To relieve a sinus headache, treat the sinus congestion as described on pages 233 to 234.

Fomentations (hot herbal compresses) can be applied to the back, neck, and shoulders to relieve the muscle tightness that contributes to stress or tension headaches. David Hoffmann recommends using hot chamomile tea for this purpose.

One of the best-known herbs for preventing migraine headache is feverfew (*Tanacetum parthenium*). Although no one has determined how feverfew interrupts migraine cycles, it is believed to contain chemicals that, like aspirin and other salicylates, block or reduce inflammatory reactions so that blood flow to the brain is not reduced. At least one double-blind, randomized, placebo-controlled, crossover trial of feverfew showed that the herb reduced both the frequency of migraine headaches and the vomiting associated with the attacks.

Herbalists familiar with feverfew recommend the following guidelines. To prevent or relieve migraine headaches, chew one or two fresh or dried leaves (if you grow the plant yourself, and if you can tolerate the taste), brew the leaves as tea (which will be bitter), swallow them with food, or take a dried feverfew capsule. The recommended daily dose of dried feverfew is about 125 milligrams. Although there is some debate about this next measurement, some researchers recommend using feverfew that contains at least 0.2 percent parthenolide.

As feverfew may cause minor side effects, its prolonged use (over four months) should be supervised by a health care professional. About 8 percent of those who take feverfew have to stop because of mouth ulcers and upset stomach. Pregnant and breast-feeding women should avoid the herb, and so should anyone taking blood-thinning medication as the combination may cause an adverse cross-reaction.

Certain aromatherapy oils, such as lavender and sandalwood, have long histories as headache therapies. In India, sandalwood paste applied to the temples is a popular treatment for headaches. You can achieve the same result by massaging a small amount of full-strength or diluted sandalwood oil into the temples at the first sign of a headache. Lavender essential oil has similar relaxing properties and is, like sandalwood essential oil, safe to apply full-strength to the skin. In his book *Advanced Aromatherapy*, Dr. Kurt Schnaubelt recommends applying a trace of melissa (lemon balm) essential oil to the temples to ease a headache. Be sure to use therapeutic quality essential oils for this purpose; see the Resources section for recommended distributors.

In *Aromatherapy for Common Ailments*, Shirley Price recommends inhaling essential oils to relieve headaches. As soon as symptoms begin, sprinkle 2 drops each of sweet marjoram, lavender, and peppermint oils on a tissue and inhale deeply three times; for a migraine, she suggests, add 1 drop of melissa (lemon balm) essential oil to the combination.

TOOTHACHES AND GUM DISEASE

As Weston Price discovered when he studied primitive tribes around the world, the traditional diets on which humans evolved generate broad jaws, and strong, healthy, perfectly aligned teeth that are free from decay.

It's impossible to recreate the world in which our ancestors lived, but by eating whole rather than processed foods, a wide variety of foods, and foods that are fresh and in season, we can do much to improve our dental health.

Bruce West, D.C., often reminds his patients and readers of his *Health Alert* newsletter that bone builds bone; that is, supplements containing raw bone help repair the skeletal system, which includes the teeth and the bones in which they are anchored. Cold-sterilized raw bone supplements also help repair damaged knees and other joints as described on pages 197 to 198. Dr. West recommends the Standard Process supplements Bio-Dent, Biost, and Calcifood Wafers in combination with a diet that is at least one-third raw to strengthen teeth, prevent receding gums, and repair all types of dental problems.

As John Ott discovered when he studied the effects of light on living organisms (see pages 16 to 18), unfiltered natural light is essential for skeletal health. Daily exposure to natural light, through open doors and windows, from shaded porches, and in outdoor activities, strengthens the entire system.

Despite the claims of America's dental associations, mercury amalgam fillings have been discredited by scientists around the world as a leading cause of serious health problems. Fortunately, the demand for holistic dental care is increasing the availability of less toxic materials and methods. Periodontal disease involves the tissues surrounding and supporting the teeth, including the gums, sockets, and periodontal membranes, which hold the teeth in their sockets. Periodontal disease includes gingivitis, which is inflammation of the gums, and periodontitis, inflammation of the periodontal membrane. Periodontal disease also includes gum abscesses or boils, which are small pockets of pus caused by tooth decay and infection. Gingivitis can be caused by infection, but it usually results from a buildup of plaque, bacteria, and food particles under and around the gums.

The symptoms of periodontal disease are pain, especially when chewing, bleeding gums, swelling, redness, halitosis (bad breath), and erosion of the bones surrounding teeth.

The medicinal properties of the neem tree have been appreciated in its native India for thousands of years. Ancient Sanskrit documents refer to the benefits of its seeds, seed oil, leaves, roots, bark, and fruits, all of which are used in traditional Ayurvedic medicine.

In India, neem twigs are toothbrushes. They are easy to use— just break off a twig, chew it, and put it to work—and their benefits include clean teeth, healthy gums, and pleasant breath. For those who use plastic toothbrushes, a drop of neem leaf tincture added to toothpaste or tooth powder provides similar benefits.

Another ancient herb with mouth care benefits is mastic, described as an ulcer cure on page 193. Mastic resin can be chewed between meals to clean the teeth, disinfect the mouth, and tone the gums. Because it improves periodontal disease, it is an ingredient in some toothpastes (see Resources).

There is no substitute for appropriate dental care when one has cavities or abscessed teeth, but pain and infection can be controlled to some extent while waiting for an appointment. Large quantities of echinacea and other infection-fighting herbs can help save teeth that were scheduled for extraction by reducing the severity of abscesses. The essential oil of cloves, a traditional remedy for tooth pain, has an anaesthetic effect, though dental researchers warn that applying full-strength clove oil to a damaged tooth can kill the tooth's nerve. Diluting clove oil in an equal amount of carrier oil reduces the risk.

The essential oil of myrrh is an ingredient in many mouthwashes. It has anti-inflammatory properties, and it helps relieve swelling and discomfort. According to Kurt Schnaubelt, rubbing niaouli essential oil on the gums strengthens them and diminishes inflammation, and the oil's antiseptic qualities protect the mouth and throat. He also recommends using it on dental floss to clean between the teeth.

Tea tree oil has similar properties, and it is such an effective essential oil for mouth care that drugstores and supermarkets carry tea tree oil toothpaste, mouthwash, dental floss, and wooden dental picks. Tea tree oil can be applied full-strength to receding or infected gums and lightly massaged with a finger or toothbrush.

Hydrosols are effective, too. "For all tooth and gum problems," says Suzanne Catty, "the hydrosol of choice is helichrysum, the Italian immortelle. Because it has the ability to regenerate cells, it helps repair receding gums, swelling, bleeding, and infection. In addition, balsam fir is a good general tonic and immune booster."

To use, Catty suggests spraying full-strength hydrosol into the mouth or pouring a small amount into a cup for use as a mouthwash. To distribute the hydrosol well, rub gently with a soft toothbrush. In addition, add the hydrosol to drinking water or tea.

If the underlying cause of a mouth problem is digestive, she recommends carrot seed or peppermint hydrosol. If an abscess is draining, bay laurel/bay leaf hydrosol combined with helichrysum hydrosol supports the lymph system as it removes infection. Where bleeding is a factor, yarrow hydrosol is effective. These same treatments improve the breath.

"Choose one or two hydrosols," she suggests, "and apply them to the affected area, and drink them throughout the day."

BURNS AND SCALDS

The first step in treating any burn or scald is to cool the skin. Immerse the burned body part in cold water, pour cold water over it, or hold ice to it. As described on page 153, essential oil cools and repairs burned skin and, if applied quickly, stops the pain on contact. So does tea tree oil. Daniel Penoel recommends a mixture of 2 to 3 parts tea tree oil to 1 part lavender essential oil. "This Franco-Australian aromatic marriage increases the power of each essential oil over what it would be when used separately," he says, adding that it is not appropriate for treating extensive or deep burns but works well for everyday burns that occur in the home. In France, green clay is a popular therapy for burns, and Dr. Penoel suggests that a small amount of essential oil be mixed with clay and water to make an effective, synergistic poultice.

When I was a child in rural northwest Oregon, pitch from fir trees was highly prized as a first-aid treatment for burns. Whenever someone was badly burned, a pitch drive would be announced in the local schools, and everyone who could collected pitch from the resin blisters of the bark of fir trees with a knife and wax paper, a sticky but wonderfully aromatic activity. The medicinal use of pitch had all but died out when it was resurrected by Forrest Smith, a retired logger from Northern California. Now his North American Tree Resin company (see Resources) is the leading source of undiluted tree resin from the pitch of Pacific coast Douglas fir, yellow pine, and other coniferous trees.

Pitch is unexcelled as a topical disinfectant. It's also sticky, which is why Smith developed PAV salve (which stands for pitch and Vaseline petroleum jelly) and lotions made of pitch and olive oil. Pitch is a specific for burns, cuts, abrasions, trauma injuries, wounds that won't heal, bacterial infections, and fungal infections such as ringworm.

Pitch should not be applied to the eyes or mucous membranes as it can be painful. Plain vegetable oil can be used to remove pitch that gets in the eyes or becomes tangled in hair, just as vegetable oil is recommended for diluting and removing essential oils that sting or burn. Some people with delicate skin may be sensitive to pitch, but dilution in olive oil makes that reaction less likely. Pitch is not recommended for internal use. Because pitch is highly flammable, it should not be used around fire or flame.

Another burn-cooling treatment is the application of a grain alcohol tincture of chamomile, calendula, comfrey, St. John's wort, or any other skin-healing herb. A man who was badly burned at an herb farm after he carelessly ignited the brush he was clearing, was treated with calendula tincture before being taken to the hospital emergency room, and by the time he arrived, his skin was already healing. The tincture had stopped the burn, removed the heat, disinfected the injury, and stimulated rapid repair.

Alternatively, make an herbal compress by soaking a thick gauze pad in aloe vera juice or gel, cool herbal tea, a tablespoon of tincture diluted in ½ cup cold water, or a full-strength hydrosol. Hold it in place with a bandage, and don't let the gauze dry out; apply more solution as needed. Cold comfrey tea is very effective; it stimulates the regeneration of damaged tissue.

After treating the burn, cover it with a generous coating of plain honey or the honey salve described below. As beekeeper Ross Conrad reported in the *Northeast Herbal Association Journal* in 1993, when honey is the only dressing, burns heal quickly and dressing changes are painless and require no scraping. Coating a burn with honey retards oxygenation by sealing the wound, which alleviates pain within seconds. Honey is hydroscopic, absorbing moisture from its surroundings, so it doesn't dry out, and its pH is too acid for bacterial growth.

Manuka honey from New Zealand has been shown to have exceptional antibiotic properties, and it is used by health care practitioners in New Zealand, Australia, and England to treat wounds, leg ulcers, burns, and eye infections. Manuka honey rated for its antibacterial activity is sold in U.S. health food stores.

Honey Burn Treatment and All-Purpose Antiseptic

To 1 cup of honey, add 1 tablespoon full strength tea tree oil, 1 teaspoon liquid grapefruit seed extract, and 1 tablespoon lavender essential oil. Stir well to mix. Store in a tightly sealed glass jar.

Note that raw honey crystallizes, forming sharp points that can injure damaged skin. Apply only liquid honey to injured skin.

Alternatively, mix 1 or 2 tablespoons of full-strength pitch with an equal amount of lavender and/or tea tree oil and add to 1 cup of pasteurized honey or a blend of honey and olive oil. This all-purpose salve is soft, easy to apply, and versatile. Use it on any burn, cut, scrape, abrasion, or infected wound.

Vitamin E is well known as a wound healer. Its application to any burn, abrasion, or cut will help prevent infection and scarring. Empty the contents of a natural vitamin E-complex capsule by pricking one end with a pin or scissor and squeezing out the oil. If desired, add liquid vitamin E to the honey salve described above.

Sunburn

The same principles described above apply to sunburn care. Cool the skin with cold water, cold tea, ice, full-strength or diluted tinctures, hydrosols, or aloe vera juice or gel. Reapply frequently.

The essential oils of lavender, peppermint, eucalyptus, chamomile, and tea tree have both cooling and skin-healing properties. Prepare a 7-percent solution as described on page 163 and spray it onto sunburned skin or apply gently with cotton.

PUNCTURE WOUNDS

Teeth, claws, thorns, splinters, and other sharp objects puncture the skin and may trap infection.

Wash the wound with plain soap and water and/or flush it with saltwater, calendula, or echinacea tincture diluted in 2 to 3 parts water; grapefruit seed extract diluted in 4 to 5 parts water; a 7-percent tea tree oil solution; a similar wash made with lavender oil; or a full strength herbal tea made with plantain, echinacea, sage, thyme, or other antiseptic, disinfecting herbs.

If available, mash a fresh plantain leaf with water to make a thick paste, mash or grind fresh wheat grass to a pulp, or mix powdered wheat grass or a similar green grass powder with water and apply the herb as a poultice. Comfrey is not recommended for puncture wounds because it heals the skin so quickly that infection may be trapped beneath the surface. Plantain and wheat grass are "drawing" herbs; they help pull embedded splinters, thorns, hair, debris, and infection from wounds. Keep the poultice or salve in place with a gauze bandage, and change it at least twice per day.

Full-strength pitch or pitch salve is an excellent treatment for puncture wounds. Simply apply and bandage.

INSECT BITES AND STINGS

Nothing neutralizes bites and stings like lavender or tea tree oil. The herbal literature is full of stories about people who saved their lives by neutralizing toxic spider bites, dangerous stings, and even some venomous snake bites with the repeated application of full-strength lavender and/or tea tree oil. Some aromatherapists use eucalyptus oil or blends of eucalyptus, lavender, and peppermint for the same purpose.

These essential oils are so widely available that it's easy to keep some on hand wherever you are. Prompt treatment interrupts swelling, itching, and pain.

Full-strength and diluted pitch has been used by physicians

and veterinarians to treat black widow and brown recluse spider bites, flea and tick bites, wasp and bee stings, poison oak and ivy rashes, and all types of injuries.

Echinacea tincture numbs the skin, disinfects the bite, and stops itching. Green clay and drawing herbs such as plantain and comfrey are effective poultices. Several years ago an unidentified spider bit my husband's hand, and within hours his hand grew hot and doubled in size while a red line began to move up his inner arm from the wrist. He refused to go to an emergency room, so I put fresh comfrey leaf and root through our wheat grass juicer, recombined the juice and pulp, covered his hand with the mixture, and tied it in place with a plastic bag and towels. The pain stopped immediately, the red line stopped growing, and the swelling began to subside. We changed the poultice twice during the night and by morning all trace of the bite had disappeared. His hand looked like a deflated balloon for a day while it recovered from its dramatic swelling, but that was the treatment's only side effect.

Any green plant can be used as an infection-drawing poultice, including wheat grass, plantain, and dandelion, but comfrey is such a powerful healer that it will always be the first choice of many herbalists.

Meat tenderizers containing papaya enzymes digest irritating proteins if applied to stings. These can be used alone or in combination with other therapies.

TRAUMA INJURIES

There are several ways to interrupt the pain, swelling, discoloration, and bruising of sharp blows to the body. One is with arnica tincture. Despite warnings to the contrary (see pages 125 to 126), full-strength arnica tincture is safe to apply to broken or bleeding skin. The more thorough and frequent the application, the faster one recovers. If applied within a minute or two of the injury, arnica can stop the pain on contact.

Dr. Penoel makes similar claims for full-strength peppermint essential oil. If applied immediately, he says, pain and swelling will stop at once. Peppermint essential oil should not be used around the eyes or mucous membranes, but it is safe to apply to bleeding wounds.

CUTS, ABRASIONS, AND INFECTED WOUNDS

Pitch, described on page 247, has significant antibacterial, antiviral, antifungal, and skin-healing properties. Applied full-strength to serious injuries, it promotes rapid and complete healing.

Forrest Smith became interested in the healing properties of pitch when he worked as a tree cutter. When a medical missionary asked for pitch to take to South America, Smith began collecting it. The physician spent several years in remote areas, where he routinely performed surgery without sterile equipment or antibiotics. Before closing every incision, he covered the area with pitch and applied more before bandaging the wound. None of his patients developed an infection and all experienced rapid healing.

Smith is fond of recounting the story of how, years ago, a friend treated a dog that had been hit by a car and lay by the side of the road with its entrails in the sand. His friend felt sorry for the dog, who was everyone's friend, so he did his best to patch him up. He had some pitch with him, so he poured it over the sandy intestines as he shoved them back into the abdominal cavity, then he covered the wound with more pitch and tied the dog together (no stitches) with bandages wrapped around his body. The dog healed completely and lived in excellent health for several more years. All of the treatments described for burns and puncture wounds can be used for cuts, abrasions, and infected wounds.

CARPAL TUNNEL SYNDROME

Also known as cumulative trauma disorder, occupational neuritis, repetitive stress injury (RSI), or overuse injury, carpal tunnel syndrome is a painful inflammation of the median nerve, which runs from the forearm to the fingertips after passing through a tunnel formed by ligaments and carpal bones in the wrist, where it controls movement of the fingers and thumbs. When the median nerve is stressed or pinched, it produces numbness, pain, or a loss of feeling in the hand.

Everyone whose work involves repetitive hand motions or twisting of the wrist is at risk, including musicians, meat cutters, carpenters, sewing machine operators, long-distance truck drivers, and operators of power tools. Many sports stress the median nerve, such as rock climbing, rowing, golf, tennis, downhill skiing, archery, and competitive shooting.

When physicians test for repetitive stress injury or carpal tunnel syndrome, they usually check for swelling, inflammation, weakness, poor reflexes, and a limited range of motion in the hand and arm. Numbness typically affects the thumb and first two fingers. Tapping the front of the wrist causes numbness in the forearm, and the Phalen wrist flexion test, also called the reverse prayer test (holding the hands together back to back, with fingers touching) produces tingling.

Dropping the hands to the sides and shaking wrists and fingers, an instinctive reaction to numbness or tingling in the hands, relieves symptoms in mild cases. Wearing an elastic wrist support or snug-fitting elastic glove helps prevent stress. In more serious cases, a wrist splint can be worn to keep the wrist from bending, especially while sleeping. Changing your hand position on the job also helps. I developed carpal tunnel syndrome several years ago while typing, but moving the computer keyboard to my lap and pressing the space bar with my index fingers instead of my thumbs has helped keep it from recurring.

There is much debate about vitamin B_6 (pyridoxine), which has brought relief to many with this disorder. When researchers found that a group of carpal tunnel syndrome patients did not share a clinical deficiency of the vitamin, they concluded that it could not alleviate the syndrome. However, numerous other studies have shown that vitamin B_6 does make a difference, so something other than a clinical vitamin B_6 deficiency may be at work. The best B-vitamin supplements are made from whole food sources and include the entire vitamin B complex, such as Standard Process Cataplex B and B-6 Niacinimide.

Massage, hydrotherapy, chiropractic, acupuncture, and other hands-on therapies are helpful, as are yoga postures that relax the back and neck.

The application of a cold pack (ice or a pack of frozen vegetables wrapped in a towel) at ten-minute intervals (ten minutes on, ten minutes off) for an hour combined with simple exercises helps relieve symptoms. Open the fingers wide and close the fist tightly a dozen times or more; tightly press fingertips together for several seconds and release, repeating twenty times or more; hold hands overhead and rotate the wrists clockwise for twenty seconds and then counterclockwise; and use a rubber grip exerciser, available in sporting goods stores and pharmacies, to strengthen hand and forearm muscles.

Cold herbal compresses and hot fomentations are also helpful. Brew a strong decoction of ginger tea by simmering 2 tablespoons powdered ginger or 4 tablespoons fresh chopped or grated gingerroot in 2 cups water for fifteen minutes. Strain half the tea into a bowl set in icewater in the sink, which will chill it quickly, and as soon as it is cool to the touch add ice cubes to make it cold. Strain the rest into a bowl and cover with a plate or saucer to retain heat. Spread a towel on a table to protect its surface, and have two hand towels and two washcloths handy.

Soak one washcloth in the hot tea, wring it out slightly, and test its temperature with your inner wrist. The tea should be hot to the touch but not scalding. If too hot for comfort, open the washcloth to release heat, and test again. Fold the washcloth in half, set it on a hand towel that you have folded in half lengthwise, rest the inner wrist on the hot washcloth, and loosely wrap the hand towel around your hand to retain heat. Holding the forearm straight to help relieve pressure, spread the fingers wide for five to ten seconds, release, and repeat several times.

After two or three minutes, the compress will have cooled. Return the washcloth to the hot tea and repeat its application.

Soak the other washcloth in the cold tea and apply a cold compress. Repeat the procedure after two or three minutes.

If both wrists are affected and you're sufficiently dexterous or have someone to help you, heat one wrist while you chill the other. Alternate the hot and cold compresses, finishing this treatment with the compress that seems to bring the most relief.

The herb turmeric has anti-inflammatory properties. Many herbalists recommend taking ½ teaspoon turmeric in capsules or mixed with water three times per day between meals. Turmeric can also be mixed with water to form a paste and applied as a poultice, but this temporarily dyes the skin yellow.

Horsetail is rich in silica, which helps build connective tissue. Horsetail tincture, capsules, and other products help repair damaged and inflamed tissue.

Ginkgo biloba, most famous as a memory tonic, increases blood circulation in the hands and wrists. Take 20 drops of tincture twice a day to help repair damage to the affected area.

While working, if possible, support the arms and elbows on a flat surface, and keep them close to the body with the wrists straight.

Whenever possible, schedule breaks in your work, such as short breaks during the day and longer breaks, such as several months, if symptoms are severe. For some, relief from carpal tunnel syndrome has come only after a career change.

Chiropractic adjustments to the neck, shoulder, elbow, and wrist often help relieve carpal tunnel syndrome. Acupuncture, acupressure, and massage are also helpful.

Repetitive motion in the legs and ankles resulting in numbness in the feet, ankles, and lower legs is called tarsal tunnel syndrome. Walking barefoot whenever possible alleviates discomfort and helps prevent the recurrence of tarsal tunnel syndrome, and so do the therapies described above.

SCIATICA

Sciatica is a painful condition caused by compression of the sciatic nerve, which extends from the base of the spine down the back of the legs to the knees, where it divides and continues on either side of the calves to the toes. At its worst, an irritated sciatic nerve causes such searing pain that the patient cannot sit, stand, walk, or move without discomfort.

Sciatica is often blamed on poor posture, muscle strain, pregnancy, obesity, wearing high heels, sleeping on a too soft mattress, or inflammation from a slipped disk or arthritis. To help prevent sciatica, most experts recommend that you sleep on a firm mattress on your back or on your side with knees bent rather than on your stomach; adjust chair height so that your feet are flat on the floor and your knees are slightly higher than your hips, or use a footrest to support and elevate your feet; avoid crossing your legs while sitting; be sure your chair has a firm back support; and, if necessary, use a pillow or cushion to help you sit with a straight back. During acute attacks, avoid lifting anything heavier than 10 pounds, push rather than pull heavy objects, and, as always, bend your legs rather than your back while lifting.

Chiropractic adjustments, especially those involving deep tissue work, help relieve pressure on the sciatic nerve.

But these are mechanical treatments for what is usually a nutritional problem, for the most common underlying cause of sciatica is a toxic colon. A lack of fresh, whole foods and the fiber they provide combined with dehydration (an insufficient consumption of plain water) and a lack of beneficial intestinal bacteria (a side effect of antibiotic drugs and a diet of processed foods) results in the accumulation of waste in the large intestine.

In his book *Acidophilus and Colon Health: The Natural Way to Prevent Disease*, David Webster describes how he woke one morning and couldn't get out of bed. The several doctors he visited were unable to alleviate his pain, but a chiropractor finally diagnosed it as a sciatic nerve attack caused by an impacted colon. She explained that the sciatic nerve, which is the largest nerve in the body, can become inflamed because of accumulated toxins, and she treated Webster with a colonic. "I walked out of her office pain-free and have never had the problem recur in the past twenty-four years," he wrote.

The famous American herbalist John R. Christopher, N.D., wrote in his classic textbook *School of Natural Healing* that toxins in the sigmoid section of the bowel irritate the sciatic nerve and help dislocate the sacroiliac. "The greatest herb for this problem," said Dr. Christopher, "is chaparral supplemented by budrock root tea." He also recommended 1 teaspoon of modified citrus pectin, which is a gentle soluble fiber, three times per day to help cleanse the intestines.

Dr. Christopher gave other suggestions, the most unusual of which is to place the right foot in a pan of chopped garlic, with the bare foot resting on the garlic, and the left foot in hot, apple cider vinegar. "This will start a circulatory movement which will give quick relief," he promised.

Systemic oral enzyme therapy (see pages 91 to 92) helps relieve sciatica. So do yoga postures that relieve constipation and pressure on the sciatic nerve, including inverted postures, and simply lying on a slant board for ten to twenty minutes once or twice a day has a similar effect.

The herb St. John's wort, which is best known for its mood-elevating properties, has long been used to heal injured nerves and sciatica. Whole-herb tinctures contain all of the herb's complex chemicals, while standardized extracts may not. One to 2 dropperfuls (up to 1 teaspoon) of whole-herb St. John's wort tincture can be taken as needed to relieve sciatica, only for a day or two. Because it does not address the underlying cause of sciatica, this herbal treatment is not a cure. Large doses of St. John's wort are not recommended for long-term use (see pages

142 to 143) or in combination with prescription or over-the-counter drugs. St John's wort oil (a massage oil made with olive oil and St. John's wort blossoms, not a distilled essential oil) can be applied to the affected area at any time; at night, this treatment helps ensure a good night's sleep.

According to Siegfried Gursche in *The Encyclopedia of Natural Healing*, a hot, stinging nettle bath is a proven remedy for acute sciatica. Soak 4 cups of dried stinging nettle leaves in a large pan of cold water for twelve hours or overnight. Heat the liquid on the stove, then strain and add it to bathwater. Sit in the tub without submerging the chest. Soak for twenty minutes and do not dry off, but put on a cotton terry bathrobe, cover yourself with blankets, and sweat in bed for one hour.

In addition, drink chamomile tea and apply chamomile tea or tincture to the affected area.

Acupuncture, massage, and other hands-on therapies help relieve sciatica. Some practitioners recommend applying heat or ice to relieve symptoms and relax tense muscles. Swimming and certain yoga postures may help release pressure on the sciatic nerve if caused by muscle spasms.

See the recommendations on pages 182 to 183 for relieving constipation, which addresses the underlying cause of sciatica.

BACK PAIN

Back pain has many causes, from pregnancy and simple muscle strain to herniated disks, kidney infections, poor posture, osteoporosis, osteoarthritis of the spine (also called spondylosis), ankylosing spondylitis (a severe form of arthritis that affects the spine), and injuries.

Obviously, treatment depends on the condition's cause. If driving long distances with a wallet in your pocket throws your hip out of alignment, curing the resulting back pain can be as easy as switching pockets.

If low back pain results from a kidney infection, medical attention is recommended. A life-threatening infection may require antibiotics, but holistic physicians treat mild kidney and bladder infections with plain water, unsweetened cranberry juice, and infection-fighting herbs like uva ursi (*Arctostaphylos uva-ursi*). Cranberry juice contains compounds that prevent bacteria from adhering to tissue lining the urinary tract, and in combination with increased quantities of plain water, it flushes bacteria and debris from the system. Uva ursi is an ingredient in many herbal kidney and bladder tonic blends.

Pregnancy causes back pain by changing a woman's center of gravity and straining muscles that support the abdomen. Obesity in both men and women causes similar problems. Strong abdominal muscles help prevent back pain by supporting internal organs and keeping the spine in its proper alignment. Athletes usually have easy, problem-free pregnancies with a minimum of discomfort, but any woman who plans to have children can minimize back pain by getting into shape and doing abdomen-strengthening exercises. If you are already pregnant, see a qualified yoga instructor, chiropractor, or personal trainer for appropriate exercises.

Arthritis causes back pain by affecting the spine itself or by disrupting the body's balance and alignment. See chapter 9 for the treatment of arthritis and related conditions.

If back pain is caused by an injury or accident, systemic oral enzyme therapy (see pages 91 to 92) and the topical application of arnica tincture (see pages 125 to 126) help remove congestion and inflammation from the area. Treating an injury with ice, such as an ice pack or bag of frozen peas, helps prevent swelling and pain.

Another helpful treatment is dimethylsulfoxide, or DMSO, which is sold in health food stores. Originally a by-product of paper manufacturing, DMSO is now produced synthetically as well as naturally for therapeutic use. In the 1960s, DMSO was tested on more than one hundred thousand patients in over three thousand published studies, all of which showed it to be safe and effective, but political pressure prevented FDA approval, which resulted in product labels that described DMSO as an industrial solvent.

"Most people have been led to believe that DMSO is nothing more than a horse liniment used by veterinarians," says David G. Williams, M.D. "Nothing could be further from the truth." Dr. Williams has used and recommended DMSO for over twenty years for arthritis, frozen shoulder, neck pain, prostate problems, tendinitis, hemorrhoids, gout, frostbite, ear problems, back pain, headaches, bursitis, phlebitis, nerve pain, tinnitus, brain damage related to stroke, joint and muscle inflammation, spider bites, trauma injuries, snoring, and diabetic polyneropathy (burning or aching pain caused by nerve damage).

According to Stanley Jacob, M.D., a professor at Oregon Health Sciences University and a leading expert on DMSO, its topical application after injury appears to reduce brain swelling and intercranial pressure. Immediate application to spinal injuries may prevent nerve damage and paralysis. DMSO's only adverse side effects are a lingering garlic fragrance on the breath and, in a few cases, minor skin irritation.

Conventional medicine used to treat injuries and chronic

back pain with prolonged bed rest, but a lack of activity actually contributes to recurring back problems. Now physicians recommend only a day or two of rest followed by increasingly vigorous daily exercise.

In fact, some medical doctors recommend no bedrest at all. No physician has so radically changed the treatment of back pain as John Sarno, M.D., professor of clinical rehabilitation medicine at New York University School of Medicine and attending physician at the Howard A. Rusk Institute of Rehabilitation Medicine, New York University Medical Center. In 1991, Dr. Sarno published *Healing Back Pain: The Mind-Body Connection*, which addressed tension myositis syndrome, or TMS, the major cause of pain in the back, neck, shoulders, buttocks, arms, and legs. An injury may trigger a physical disorder, says Dr. Sarno, but it is the mind that causes ongoing pain in muscles, nerves, tendons, and ligaments. He suggests stopping all medication, physical therapy, and treatments that focus on symptoms, and replacing them with the realization that suppressed emotions are the actual cause of physical discomfort.

Many of Sarno's patients are veterans of both conventional and alternative therapies, having undergone back surgery, physical therapy, chiropractic, and other treatments with little or no improvement. His treatment for all is a group lecture explaining why conventional therapy doesn't work and telling patients to resume their normal activities without thinking about conventional medical wisdom or the details of their injuries. Instead, he tells them, get in touch with underlying anger, anxiety, frustration, guilt, depression, low self-esteem, and similar emotions, to which he attributes disorders as varied as back pain, neck and hand pain, herniated discs, carpal tunnel syndrome, fibromyalgia, repetitive strain injuries, migraine headaches, hay fever, colitis, ulcers, and even acne. His treatment plan includes meditation and sometimes psychotherapy, including behavior modification, but its most important component is the patient's realization that it is the mind, not the body, that causes pain.

Along more conventional lines, back pain often improves as a result of hands-on therapies (see chapter 12). In addition, herbs, essential oils, and hydrosols that help muscles relax, such as chamomile and lavender, are effective teas, compresses, massage oil ingredients, and aromatherapy treatments. The topical application of comfrey as a poultice or compress (see page 264) has helped many back injuries heal in record time.

In the 1950s, an osteopath demonstrated to football coach and trainer H. Meares a simple way to relieve his players' back and hip pain. A player would lie on his back while the trainer held his hand under the player's sacrum for twenty minutes. Elevating the sacrum in this manner helped tight muscles relax, allowing the spine to return to its proper alignment. The trainer then taped the player's hips tightly to stabilize his hips and sacrum.

The success of this simple therapy led to development of the Sacro Wedgy and Sacro Hip Belt (see Resources), which have helped patients with sciatica, herniated disks, back pain associated with pregnancy, and injuries common to runners, golfers, and other athletes.

Chiropractors routinely adjust the spine and joints to bring the body into balance, and several yoga postures help improve balance and alignment. There are so many possible cures for acute or chronic back pain that just about anyone who explores alternative therapies should be able to find lasting relief without the use of prescription drugs or surgery.

BONE SPURS

Abnormal growth at the ends of bones, especially in the spine and extremities, can interfere with nerves and muscles during normal activity by causing sharp or excruciating pain.

Bone spurs often develop at the base of the heel, where they result from stress that causes the heel bone to develop a knobby protrusion. When they occur in the spine, bone spurs cause back or neck pain. In some cases, bone spurs occur in the hand.

One possible cause of bone spurs is insufficient or insufficiently absorbed calcium. Some experts blame milk and other dairy products for the development of bone spurs because the minerals in milk are often poorly assimilated (see pages 80 to 84).

Some health care practitioners blame inadequate hydrochloric acid production (see pages 86 to 88) and the use of over-the-counter antacid products for the impaired absorption of calcium and other minerals. In addition to avoiding products that suppress or neutralize hydrochloric acid, consider taking enzymes with food and between meals (see page 91) to improve digestion and remove toxins from the system.

Food-source supplements that provide calcium, magnesium, boron, silicon, sulfur, manganese, zinc, copper, and vitamin D are recommended to help prevent the development of bone spurs.

The most effective herb for this condition may be comfrey, also known as knit bone, which can be applied as a poultice over the affected area as well as taken internally. Dr. John Christopher was famous for his "Regeneration Tea," which he made using 6 parts comfrey root (*Symphytum officinale*), 6 parts oak bark (*Quercus robur*), 3 parts gravel root (*Eupatorium purpureum*), 3 parts mullein (*Verbascum thapsus*), 1 part lobelia (*Lobelia inflata*), 2 parts wormwood (*Artemisia absinthium*), 3 parts marshmallow root (*Althea officinalis*), 1 part skullcap (*Scutellaria laterifolia*), and 3 parts walnut bark (*Juglans regia*). To brew, mix 1 gallon filtered, distilled, or spring water with 1 cup loose tea in a stainless steel or enamel pot and let stand overnight. Heat the tea, let it simmer without boiling for twenty minutes, and strain through cheesecloth or a stainless steel strainer. After straining, heat the tea and simmer it down to half its original volume.

Refrigerate the tea in glass jars and use as needed. In a 1993 report on bone regeneration, health newsletter publisher Sam Biser documented with photographs several cases in which people who learned of Dr. Christopher's formula used it to heal their bone spurs, shattered kneecaps, broken backs, severed tendons, tennis elbow, crushed toes, fractured hips, and other injuries. In one case, a five-year-old boy whose hand was injured in a car accident reportedly regrew three fingers that were severed at the knuckle after several months of treatment with hot, comfrey-lobelia compresses. A woman who reported having a large bone spur in her hand used the tea as a compress, and after five months of daily application, it disappeared.

The tea can be used to soak a fracture, injury, or bone spur in the hands or feet. It can be used to soak cotton towels or cheesecloth to make a compress, which is held in place with plastic or fabric. A woman who lost most of her kneecap in an accident mixed the tea with clay to make a poultice that she held in place overnight with plastic and toweling, and rinsed it off the next morning. She did this six nights per week, and within six months her kneecap was completely restored. Conventional Western medicine does not accept claims that human body parts can regenerate, but to practitioners of traditional herbal medicine, such reports are realistic and accurate. Readers are invited to contact Sam Biser (see Resources) and the people whose stories he published.

Because of comfrey's controversial alkaloids (see notes on comfrey's safety, pages 128 to 130), some herbalists recommend replacing it with other herbs. Unfortunately, no other herbs work as well. To ensure safety, take liver-protecting herbs like dandelion or milk thistle seed at the same time, use comfrey externally while leaving it out of teas made for drinking, or take a comfrey tincture from which potentially harmful alkaloids have been removed (see Resources).

EARACHES

Pain in the ears can be caused by an infection, injury, a ruptured eardrum, the presence of a foreign object such as a seed, insect, or ear plug, excessive earwax that has hardened in the outer ear canal, changes in atmospheric pressure during flying, tooth problems, or temporomandibular joint syndrome (TMJ).

Some of these conditions, such as foreign objects in the ear, an abscessed tooth, or mastoiditis (a serious infection that causes the discharge of thick pus from the ear), require immediate medical attention.

But some causes of ear pain can be treated at home with excellent results. Many parents become interested in medicinal herbs after antibiotics fail to cure their children's ear infections. An herbal ear oil made with olive oil, mullein blossoms, and/or garlic often succeeds where antibiotics fail—and without the drugs' expense or adverse side effects. Several popular ear oils are sold in health food stores, or make your own as described on page 149.

Swimmer's ear is an infection caused by bacteria or fungi that thrive in the damp, warm, dark ear canal, causing itching, dull pain that worsens when the earlobe is pulled, and in some cases fever and temporary hearing loss. Conventional medicine treats swimmer's ear with painkillers, antibiotics, and antifungal drugs along with the advice to keep the ears dry for several weeks. Alternatives to prescription drugs include infection-fighting herbs like echinacea, which can be taken in capsules, tea, or tinctures, and garlic, which can be taken as aged garlic extract or fresh garlic added to food. The same ear oil that treats childhood ear infections helps prevent swimmer's ear.

Other first-aid measures include placing a hot comfrey tea bag (steeped and strained) on the ear to help alleviate pain and inflammation, taking an echinacea-goldenseal tincture according to label directions to help fight infection, applying ear drops that contain grapefruit seed extract or tea tree oil to reduce bacteria and fungi, rinsing the ears with warm chamomile tea, and avoiding dairy products, which often contribute to ear infections.

When ear pain is caused by excessive or hardened wax in the ears, daily applications of warmed olive oil or herbal ear oil help relieve the condition. Another effective treatment is the use of ear candles, a traditional Asian remedy now popular in Germany, India, Egypt, Japan, Australia, and North America. In this two-person procedure, a hollow ear candle is placed in the outer ear canal and its opposite end is lit. Most ear candles sold in American health food stores are made of unbleached cotton or linen soaked in hot paraffin or beeswax, and some contain herbs or essential oils. According to Russell Sheppard in his *Practical Guide to Ear Candling*, the burning candle creates a gentle, soft flow of warmth and smoke that flows into the ear, drying it out, softening earwax, and relieving discomfort. An aluminum pie plate is held between the patient's head and the flame, which is extinguished as soon as it comes within four inches of the ear. Although some users confuse the burned candle's waxy residue with earwax, says Sheppard, ear candles do not remove wax from the ear. Instead, the process softens earwax, allowing the ear to excrete wax and other material for a few days after the procedure.

Some users report improved hearing, relief from sinus and allergy symptoms, reduced ringing, buzzing, or itching of the ears, or headache relief after one or several candling sessions. For information, suppliers, and detailed instructions, see the Resources section.

CHAPTER TWELVE

So Many Choices

ONE REASON THE ALTERNATIVE or complementary therapy marketplace is confusing is that there are so many choices. As the preceding chapters explain, there are dozens of ways to treat and prevent chronic and acute conditions with do-it-yourself nutritional and herbal therapies. In addition, health care practitioners offer a variety of professional services, which are growing in popularity because they are nontoxic, drug-free, and not invasive.

One of the most familiar and well-established alternative therapies in America is chiropractic. Chiropractic doctors, who use the initials D.C. after their names, examine the body's bones, muscles, ligaments, and tendons in order to diagnose and treat disorders associated with the musculo-skeletal and nervous systems. Subluxations, or misalignments of vertebrae in the spine, interfere with good health by affecting posture, restructuring movement of the ribs, causing neck muscles to contract, producing muscle spasm, interrupting the normal flow of energy through nerves, and affecting the function of glands and organs.

One type of chiropractic adjustment involves the stretching of a joint just beyond its normal range of motion, producing an audible, painless click. Another uses gentle touch along the spine, skull, and pelvis. Other adjustments are more vigorous. Direct thrust techniques or high-velocity thrusts can be accompanied by a loud cracking noise. Some chiropractors use a hand-held instrument that gently repositions vertebrae, or they may combine the adjustment of subluxations with other therapies, such as the application of heat, cold, ultrasound, electrical stimulation, massage, nutrition, and exercise.

Although most people associate chiropractic adjustment with back pain, skilled chiropractors treat every structural problem from headaches to sciatica, sports injuries, and respiratory problems such as asthma. Even some case of female infertility can be treated with chiropractic adjustments of the pelvis.

In addition to making skeletal adjustments, some chiropractors release tension and pain from muscles with deep tissue or trigger-point work, which involves pressing muscles at intervals along the body.

This approach to pain relief was pioneered by Janet Travell, M.D. (the personal physician of President John F. Kennedy), and Raymond Nimmo, D.C., a Texas chiropractor. Working independently, both concluded that pain which is not caused by illness but which occurs in otherwise healthy joints is caused by trigger points in the muscles and connective tissue. Using finger pressure similar to that of shiatsu massage or acupressure, the therapist presses deeply into painful areas, stretching muscles and connective tissue. Releasing the pressure causes tightened muscles to relax, allowing the release of waste products that are trapped in the trigger points.

Dr. Travell treated trigger points by injecting them with saline, a salt solution, and procaine, a local anaesthetic. Her work was expanded by Bonnie Prudden, who discovered that deep pressure applied for five to seven seconds relieved pain without the need for injections. Prudden developed a system of trigger-point massage called myotherapy.

Dr. Nimmo developed a chiropractic protocol known as Receptor-Tonus Technique, which "triggers" muscle nerve receptors to affect the tone or tension of muscles. Some practitioners use a spray-and-stretch technique in which a cooling spray is applied to muscles to desensitize stretch inhibitors, allowing muscles to be fully stretched, or they may apply concentrated moist heat or ultrasound. All these techniques decrease pain, restore normal muscle motion, and relieve pressure on joints under affected muscles.

Another system that uses press-and-release motion is reflexology, which evolved from a European system called zone therapy. Reflexology maps of the hands and feet show their connections to other parts of the body. The pads of the toes correspond to the sinuses, brain, and head area, while the arch of the foot represents the lower digestive tract, and the upper part of the heel corresponds to the sciatic nerve. All the glands and organs, including the eyes and ears, are represented by other parts of the foot. Similarly, the pads of the fingertips represent the sinuses, the base of the palm represents the lower digestive tract, and the inner wrist corresponds to the lower lumbar region.

Practitioners of reflexology massage the feet or hands and stimulate the different zones with finger pressure or with the application of wooden tools or other objects. Tender or painful areas are believed to be congested or blocked. "If it hurts," say reflexologists, "work it out." The stimulation of reflex points helps release blocked energy, thus improving the functioning of glands, organs, and other body parts.

Experienced reflexologists have helped treat all types of painful conditions, including asthma, indigestion, headache, sore throat, anxiety, backache, head colds, menstrual problems, and injuries. Mildred Carter's popular book *Hand Reflexology* describes specific treatments for more than a hundred conditions, including toothache and anemia. Her book even includes letters from people who treated their dogs for asthma and other conditions by massaging their paws.

Osteopathy, a system of whole-body healing, was developed in 1870 by Andrew Taylor Still, an army surgeon originally trained as an engineer. His system of adjusting the body relieves muscle strain and correctly positions misaligned bones, thus encouraging the body to heal from within. Osteopaths use the abbreviation D.O. (Doctor of Osteopathy) after their names. Soft tissue manipulation, gentle head adjustments called cranial osteopathy, and other techniques allow osteopaths to treat joint and muscle pain, backache, neck problems, sciatica, injuries, headaches, and other conditions.

Chiropractic, trigger-point work, reflexology, and osteopathic therapies were developed only recently. Far older are the treatments used in traditional Oriental medicine (TOM) or traditional Chinese medicine (TCM). Medical doctors trained in China, Tibet, and other Asian countries often use the title Doctor of Oriental Medicine (DOM) or Licensed Acupuncturist (L.Ac.) when they move to the United States.

In traditional Oriental or Chinese medicine, everything depends on the flow of chi. Also spelled qi and pronounced "chee," chi is the invisible life force that circulates through every living being. Modern researchers describe chi in terms of electromagnetic energy. It flows through the body along lines or channels called meridians, each of which is associated with a gland or organ. Practitioners of traditional Oriental medicine use pulse diagnosis and other means of determining whether a patient's chi is flowing freely. Blocked chi creates imbalances that lead to illness. Treatment that releases blockages and enhance the circulation of chi include acupuncture, acupressure, shiatsu massage, energy work such as qi gong, dietary changes, lifestyle changes, and the use of medicinal herbs. Tai chi, a gentle exercise of dancelike movements requiring focus and concentration, is said to stimulate the flow of chi and improve health.

In acupuncture, the practitioner inserts thin, sterile needles at appropriate acupuncture points to free blockages and stimulate the flow of chi. This ancient therapy is best known for its effect on pain. In China, acupuncture has been used as an anesthetic, allowing patients to remain conscious during surgery. In the United States, muscle and joint conditions such as back pain, trauma injuries, bursitis, and arthritis are the most commonly treated conditions. It has also been shown to reduce the pain of childbirth and help repair the damage caused by strokes. The journal *Neurology* recently reported that acupuncture improved mobility and balance, shortened recovery time, and enhanced the long-term independence of stroke victims. In addition, it often helps relieve depression, anxiety, fatigue, and allergies.

The World Health Organization (WHO) recognizes the use of acupuncture in the treatment of a wide range of medical problems as well as physical problems related to stress and illness. Acupuncture has been shown to reduce withdrawal symptoms in those giving up cigarettes, alcohol, and addictive drugs.

Shiatsu massage and acupressure are often called acupuncture without needles, for they stimulate acupuncture points with physical pressure, releasing the flow of chi through the body's energy channels. Acupressure usually involves the thumbs and fingers, while shiatsu practitioners use their hands, knees, and elbows. Both therapies free energy blockages along the same meridians used by acupuncture.

Shiatsu is only one type of massage. Many schools or systems of massage have developed around the world, but most involve manipulation of the body's muscles, ligaments, and tendons with long and short strokes, kneading, wringing, squeezing, pummeling, and pressing soft tissue with the thumbs, fingers, or knuckles. Massage relaxes muscles, stimulates circulation, increases the flow of lymph, speeds the healing of sports injuries, and relieves pain. In addition to improving such conditions as arthritis, rheumatism, and sciatica, massage can relieve headaches, improve digestion, relieve constipation, alleviate premenstrual tension, and reduce anxiety. Massage can also help reduce swelling from fractures, improve wound healing, break up scar tissue, improve the mobility of muscles affected by old injuries, promote the drainage of sinus fluids, and help relieve insomnia.

Other types of bodywork include the Feldenkrais method, which replaces old patterns of movement with new ones so effectively that paralyzed muscles can be taught to move; Rolfing, a system of manual manipulation that corrects posture and relieves pain; Hellerwork, which teaches people to sit, stand, lift, run, and walk more efficiently; the Trager approach, in which practitioners use rocking, pulling, and rotational movements to relieve tension and stiffness of the head, torso, arms, and legs; and the Alexander technique, a process of reeducation that uses posture to improve freedom of movement and the efficient use of the body.

Homeopathy, still another system of medicine, was developed in the early 1800s by the German physician Samuel Hahnemann. He wrote, "If a medicine administered to a healthy person causes a certain syndrome of symptoms, that medicine will cure a sick person who presents similar symptoms." Hahnemann believed that these medicines, taken in dilute form, cause the body to heal itself. The basis of his principle is "like cures like"—for example, a substance that causes a fever in a healthy person will cure a fever in someone who is ill.

Despite a widespread belief to the contrary, homeopathic drugs are not the same as herbal teas and tinctures. Medicinal herbs are used in homeopathy, but their extreme dilution makes the resulting drug very different from a standard herbal preparation. Homeopathic drugs are made from vegetable, mineral, animal, and other sources. These are first made into a crude substance or tincture, which is then diluted several times, and each dilution is vigorously shaken or succussed. Dr. Hahnemann discovered that this method of diluting and succussing increases a medicine's curative powers while reducing the likelihood of undesirable side effects.

Substances that are not soluble in water or alcohol are triturated, that is, ground to a powder using mortar and pestle, then diluted with milk sugar. Once a substance is diluted in milk sugar in a one part per million ratio, it is considered soluble in water or alcohol. With each step, the liquid is diluted by a factor of 100, and the mixture is subjected to a series of sharp succussions, shakes, or poundings. In Hahnemann's day, the work was all done by hand; today it is partly mechanized, but long trituration and succussion are still considered necessary.

Homeopathic medicines are available in several forms. A mother tincture is an alcohol extract of the original substance, such as an undiluted herbal tincture. These are generally used for external application, as arnica tincture is used to treat bruises, but their main use is as ingredients of homeopathic drugs. Triturations are powders, or tablets made of powder, consisting of the original substance finely ground and mixed with milk sugar. These may be taken by mouth, held under the tongue until dissolved, or diluted in distilled water. Tablets are sugar tablets that contain drops of a liquid remedy.

The potency of homeopathic medicines is measured according to the number of dilutions it has undergone. The highest homeopathic potencies, which are the most diluted, are considered the strongest. The alleged power of such extremely dilute solutions is one of the paradoxes of homeopathic medicine.

Like chiropractic, therapeutic massage, acupuncture, and the other disciplines mentioned in this chapter, homeopathy is most effective when administered by an experienced practitioner. All these therapies are explained in magazines, videotapes, audiotapes, and books available in bookstores, libraries, and health food stores. In most U.S. cities, holistic health organizations publish directories of local practitioners and their specialties; check with your local health food store or library for referrals.

Bibliography

ACCIARDO, MARCIA MADHURI. *Light Eating for Survival.*
Fairfield, Iowa: 21st Century Publications, 1977.
ATKINS, ROBERT. *Dr. Atkins' New Diet Revolution.* New York:
Avon Books, 1992.
BALCH, JAMES F. and PHYLLIS A. BALCH. *Prescription for Nutri-
tional Healing.* Garden City Park, N.Y.: Avery Publishing
Group, 1990.
BATMANGHELIDJ, FEREYDOON. *Your Body's Many Cries for
Water.* Falls Church, Va.: Global Health Solutions, 1992.
BRADFORD, NIKKI, ed. *The One Spirit Encyclopedia of Comple-
mentary Health.* London: Hamlyn, 1996.
BROOKS, LINDA. *Rebounding to Better Health: A Practical Guide
to the Ultimate Exercise.* Albuquerque, N.Mex.: KE Publish-
ing, 1995.
BUCHMAN, DIAN DINCIN. *Herbal Medicine.* New York:
Random House, 1996.
BURTON GOLDBERG GROUP. *Alternative Medicine: The
Definitive Guide.* Tiburon, Calif.: Future Publishing, 1994.
CARTER, ALBERT E. *The New Miracles of Rebound Exercise.*
Fountain Hills, Ariz.: ALM Publishers, 1988.
CARTER, MILDRED, ET. AL. *Hand Reflexology: Key to Perfect
Health.* Upper Saddle River, N.J.: Prentice Hall, 2000.

CHRISTOPHER, JOHN. *School of Natural Healing*. Springville, Utah: Christopher Publications, 1976.

COCA, ARTHUR M. *The Pulse Test: The Secret of Building Your Basic Health*. New York: St. Martin's Press, 1996.

COLBIN, ANNEMARIE. *Food and Healing*. New York: Random House, 1986 and 1996.

D'ADAMO, PETER J. *Eat Right 4 Your Type*. New York: Berkeley Books, 1997.

DIAMOND, HARRY and MARILYN DIAMOND. *Fit for Life*. New York: Warner Books, 1987.

ENIG MARY. *Know Your Fats: The Complete Primer for Understanding the Nutrition of Fats, Oils, and Cholesterol*. Bethesda, Md.: Bethesda Press, 2000.

ERASMUS, UDO. *Fats That Heal, Fats That Kill*. Burnaby, B.C., Canada: Alive Books, 1993.

FALLON, SALLY and MARY ENIG. *Nourishing Traditions: The Cookbook that Challenges Politically Correct Nutrition and Diet Dictocrats*, 2d. ed. Washington, D.C.: New Trends Publishing, 1999.

FISCHER, WILLIAM L. *How to Fight Cancer and Win*. Burnaby, B.C., Canada: Alive Books, 1988.

GITTLEMAN, ANN LOUISE. *Beyond Pritikin*. New York: Bantam Books, 1998.

GLADSTAR, ROSEMARY. *Herbal Healing for Women*. New York: Simon & Schuster, 1993.

GOLOS, N. and F. GOLBITZ. *If This Is Tuesday, It Must Be Chicken: Or How to Rotate Your Food for Better Nutrition*. Los Angeles: Keats Publishing, 1983.

GOTTSCHALL, ELAINE. *Breaking the Vicious Cycle: Intestinal Health Through Diet*. Baltimore, Ontario, Canada: Kirkton Press, Ltd., 1994.

GURSCHE, SIEGFRIED, ET AL. *The Encyclopedia of Natural Healing, A Practical Self-Help Guide.* Burnaby, B.C., Canada: Alive Publishing, 1998.

HerbalGram. See American Botanical Council in the Resources section.

The Herb Companion. Herb Companion Press, P.O. Box 55295, Boulder, Colo. 80322-5295. Phone: 1-800-456-5835, www.interweave.com.

The Herb Quarterly. Long Mountain Press, Inc., 223 San Anselmo Avenue, Suite 7, San Anselmo, Calif. 94960.

HOFFMANN, DAVID. *An Elder's Herbal.* Rochester, Vt.: Healing Arts Press, 1993.

———. *Natural Relief from Headaches, Insomnia & Stress.* Los Angeles: Keats Publishing, 1999.

HOWELL, EDWARD. *Enzyme Nutrition: The Food Enzyme Concept.* Garden City Park, N.Y.: Avery Publishing Group, 1985.

KUSHIO, MICHIO. *Natural Healing Through Macrobiotics.* Tokyo and New York: Japan Publications, 1984.

LAWLESS, JULIA. *The Encyclopedia of Essential Oils.* Dorset, England and Rockport, Mass.: Element Books Limited, 1992.

LEY, BETH M. *Dr. John Willard's Catalyst Altered Water.* Fargo, N.Dak.: Christopher Lawrence Communications, 1990.

LOES, MICHAEL. *The Aspirin Alternative.* Freedom Press, 1999.

LUST, JOHN. *The Herb Book.* New York: Bantam Books, 1974.

MCCALAB, ROBERT S., EVELYN LEIGH, and KRISTA MORIEN. *Encyclopedia of Popular Herbs.* Roseville, Calif.: Prima Health, 2000.

NEWMARK, THOMAS M. and PAUL SCHULICK. *Beyond Aspirin: Nature's Answer to Arthritis, Cancer, and Alzheimer's Disease.* Prescott, Ariz.: Hohm Press, 2000.

ORNISH, DEAN. *Dr. Dean Ornish's Program for Reversing Heart Disease.* New York: Random House, 1990.

OSKI, FRANK. *Don't Drink Your Milk: New Frightening Medical Facts about the World's Most Overrated Nutrient.* Brushton, N.Y.: Teacher Services, 1992.

OTT, JOHN. *Health and Light.* Columbus, Ohio: Ariel Press, 1976.

PDR for Herbal Medicines. Montvale, N.J.: Medical Economics Company, 2000.

PENOEL, DANIEL and ROSE-MARIE PENOEL. *Natural Home Health Care Using Essential Oils.* Hurricane, Utah: Essential Science Publishing, 1998.

PESKIN, BRIAN. *Beyond the Zone.* Houston, Tex.: Noble Publishing, 2000.

PRICE, SHIRLEY. *Aromatherapy for Common Ailments.* New York: Simon & Schuster, 1991.

PRICE, WESTON. *Nutrition and Physical Degeneration: A Comparison of Primitive and Modern Diets and Their Effects.* La Mesa, Calif.: Price-Pottenger Foundation, 1945.

PRITIKIN, NATHAN. *Live Longer Now.* New York: Bantam Books, 1974.

POTTENGER, FRANCIS M., JR. *Pottenger's Cats: A Study in Nutrition.* La Mesa, Calif.: Price-Pottenger Nutrition Foundation, 1983.

REILLY, HAROLD J. and RUTH HAGY BROD. *The Edgar Cayce Handbook for Health through Drugless Therapy.* Virginia Beach, Va.: ARE Press, 1975.

SARNO, JOHN. *Healing Back Pain: The Mind-Body Connection.* New York: Warner Books, 1991.

———. *Mind Over Back Pain: A Radically New Approach to the Diagnosis and Treatment of Back Pain.* New York: Berkeley Publishing Group, 1999.

————. *The Mind-Body Prescription: Healing the Pain*. New York: Warner Books, 1999.

SCHNAUBELT, KURT. *Advanced Aromatherapy: The Science of Essential Oil Therapy*. Translated from the German by Michael Beasley. Rochester, Vt.: Healing Arts Press, 1998.

SCHOENECK, ANNELIES. *Making Sauerkraut and Pickled Vegetables at Home: The Original Lactic Acid Fermentation Method*. Burnaby, B.C., Canada: Alive Books, 1988.

SHEPPARD, RUSSELL. *Practical Guide to Ear Candling*. Auburn, Calif.: Wally's Natural Products, 1999.

TREBEN, MARIA. *Health through God's Pharmacy: Advice and Experiences with Medicinal Herbs*. Rochester, Vt.: Healing Arts Press, 1988.

WALKER, MORTON. *Jumping for Health: A Guide to Rebounding Aerobics*. Garden City Park, N.Y.: Avery Publishing Group 1989.

WALKER, NORMAN. *DMSO: Nature's Healer*. Garden City Park, N.Y.: Avery Publishing Group, 1992.

WEBSTER, DAVID. *Acidophilus and Colon Health: The Natural Way to Prevent Disease*. Cardiff, Calif.: Hygeia Publishing, 1995.

WEIL, ANDREW, M.D. *Spontaneous Healing: How to Discover and Enhance Your Body's Natural Ability to Maintain and Heal Itself*. New York: Fawcett Columbine, 1995.

WIGMORE, ANN. *The Hippocrates Diet and Health Program*. Garden City Park, N.Y.: Avery Publishing Group, 1984.

WOLCOTT, WILLIAM. *The Metabolic Typing Diet*. New York: Doubleday, 2000.

WORWOOD, VALERIE ANN. *The Complete Book of Essential Oils & Aromatherapy*. London: Macmillan London Limited, 1990; San Rafael, Calif.: New World Library, 1991.

Resources

The addresses, telephone numbers, fax numbers, and Internet websites listed here are subject to change. Your public library's reference librarian can help you locate publishers and manufacturers that have moved or whose area codes have changed since this book went to press.

SIMPLE, HOLISTIC WAYS TO IMPROVE YOUR HEALTH

Aspartame Consumer Safety Network
P.O. Box 780634
Dallas, TX 75379
Phone: 1-800-969-6050
    Distributes *Deadly Deception: The Story of Aspartame* by Mary Nash Stoddard and "The Aspartame Conspiracy," a video documentary.

Linda Brooks, Certified Reboundologist
750 Boyce Street
Urbana, OH 43078
Phone: 937-484-8206
E-mail: reboundvy@aol.com
    Nedak rebounders, instruction videos, books.

Duro-Test Corporation
9 Law Drive
Fairfield, NJ 07007
Phone: 1-800-289-3876
Vita-Lite full-spectrum fluorescent tubes. Of all the fluorescent and incandescent lights that are advertised as full-spectrum, this brand, while not a replacement for natural sunlight, may have fewer deficiencies than other fluorescents.

Eden Foods
701 Tecumseh Road
Clinton, MI 49236
Phone: 1-800-248-0301 or 517-456-7424
Fax: 517-456-6075
Imports Eden brand unrefined, sun-dried Atlantic sea salt from France. Sold in health food stores.

Gold Mine Natural Food Company
3419 Hancock Street
San Diego, CA 92110-4307
Phone: 1-800-475-FOOD
Fax: 619-296-9756
Imports unrefined sea salt from France and Mexico. Mail order.

Grain and Salt Society
273 Fairway Drive
Asheville, NC 28805
Phone: 1-800-867-7258 or 704-299-9005
Fax: 704-299-1640

Imports unrefined Celtic sea salt from France, including Flower of the Ocean, the world's finest and most expensive salt. Mail order.

Lima nv
Industrielaan 11a
9990 Maldegem, Belgium
Phone: 1-800-400-5462
Exports Lima unrefined sea salt from France. Sold in health food stores.

NatureWorks, a division of ABKIT, Inc.
New York, NY 10128
Swedish Bitters dry herbs in 30-gram boxes. Sold in health food stores. For best results, follow package directions when combining herbs and vodka, but instead of straining after eight to fourteen days as recommended, let stand six weeks or longer.

Richters Herbs
Goodwood, Ontario, L0C 1A0, Canada
Phone: 905-640-6677
Fax: 905-640-6641
E-mail: orderdesk@richters.com.
Flora Swedenbitters (Swedish Bitters dry herbs) in 35-gram packages. Mail order. See note under NatureWorks, above.

FOOD AS MEDICINE

Home Cure
P.O. Box 41420
Mesa, AZ 85274
Phone: 1-800-559-2873 or 480-443-3373
   Sweet Balance sugar-free, no-calorie sweetener made
from kiwi fruit.

Metabolic Typing Educational Center
Phone: 650-325-1840
www.metaboliced.com
   Educational and metabolic typing services affiliated
with William Wolcott.

North American Pharmacal, Inc.
17 High Street
Norwalk, CT 06851
Phone: 1-877-ABO-TYPE or 203-866-7664
Fax: 203-838-4066
www.4yourtype.com
   Home blood-type test.

Personalized Metabolic Nutrition
520 Tamalpais Drive, Suite 206
Corte Madera, CA 94925
Phone: 415-924-1471
Fax: 415-927-4664
www.bloodph.com
   Metabolic typing self-test for home use.

Right Products Company
22 High Street
Brattleboro, VT 05301
Phone: 1-800-543-7279
Home blood-type test.

CREATING THE CUSTOM DIET

Advanced Nutrition Products
P.O. Box 1634
Rockville, MD 20850
Phone: 1-888-436-7200
Fax: 301-963-3886
ImmunoGuard brand lactoferrin, Oralmat rye grass
extract.

Alive Books
7436 Fraser Park Drive
Burnaby, BC V5J 5B9
Phone: 1-800-663-6580 or 604-419-5017
Book and magazine publisher.

Bernard Jensen Products
P.O. Box 8
Solana Beach, CA 92075
Sweet whey and other products, distributed through
health food stores.

Bioforce of America
P.O. Box 507
Kinderhook, NY 12106
Phone: 518-758-6060
Imports Molkosan concentrated whey. Sold in health food stores.

A Campaign for Real Milk
Sponsored by the Weston A. Price Foundation
PMB 106-380
4200 Wisconsin Avenue, NW
Washington, DC 20016
www.realmilk.com
Grassroots organization campaigning for the return of raw, unpasteurized, unhomogenized, whole milk from organically raised, grass-fed dairy cattle.

Deep Root Organic
P.O. Box 100
Westminster Station, VT 05159
Phone: 802-722-9203
Fax: 802-722-4211
Distributes lacto-fermented sauerkraut, carrots, red cabbage, and beets.

Essential Oil Company
1719 S.E. Umatilla Street
Portland, OR 97202
Phone: 1-800-729-5912
Fax: 503-872-8767
www.essentialoil.com

Organic hand-pressed, unprocessed coconut oil from Jamaica. Mail order.

Flora, Inc.
Lynden, WA 98264
Phone: 1-800-446-2110
www.florainc.com
Udo's Choice Perfected Oil Blend, superior-quality EFA blend. Sold in health food stores.

Gold Mine Natural Food Company
3419 Hancock Street
San Diego, CA 92110-4307
Phone: 1-800-475-FOOD
Fax: 619-296-9756
Japanese salad presses and organic foods by mail.

International Yogurt Company
628 N. Doheny Drive
Los Angeles, CA 90069
Supplies health food stores with kefir grains, yogurt starter, and yogurt supplements.

Jay Robb Enterprises, Inc.
1530 Encinitas Boulevard
Encinitas, CA 92024
Phone: 1-877-529-7622
Fax: 760-634-5490
ProFlora sweet whey.

LabOne, Inc.
10101 Renner Boulevard
Lenexa, KS 66219
Phone: 913-888-1770
Fax: 913-888-0771
Inexpensive vitamin D blood test; locations nationwide.
See Krispin Sullivan, C.N., for supplement protocols.

Lactaid
P.O. Box 11
Pleasantville, NJ 08232
Lactaid milk-digesting enzyme and Beano legume-digesting enzyme products. Sold in supermarkets and health food stores.

Natural Lifestyle Supply Company
16 Lookout Drive
Asheville, NC 28804-3330
Phone: 1-800-752-2775
German pickle crocks, Japanese salad presses, and organic foods by mail.

New England Cheesemaking Supply Company
P.O. Box 65
Ashfield, MA 01330
Phone: 413-628-3808
Kefir culture, Bulgarian yogurt culture, and several cheese starter cultures.

Nutri–Health Products
218 Justin Drive
Cottonwood, AZ 86326
Phone: 1–800–362–0168
Flora Source probiotic capsules contain fourteen
strains of beneficial bacteria, including acidophilus.

Piima
P.O. Box 2614
La Mesa, CA 91943
Piima culture makes fermented dairy products. Send a
check for $5 for one package or $20 for five with name
and address. Detailed instructions for making butter,
cream cheese, whey, and other dairy products with piima
are published in *Nourishing Traditions* by Sally Fallon.

Price–Pottenger Nutrition Foundation
7890 Broadway
Lemongrove, CA 91845
Phone: 1–800–355–3748
Fax: 619–462–7600
E-mail: info@price-pottenger.org
Organization devoted to the discoveries of anthropolo-
gist/dentist Weston A. Price and nutritional physician
Francis Pottenger, Jr.

The Sprout House
17267 Sundance Drive
Ramona, CA 92065
Phone: 1–800–SPROUTS
www.sprouthouse.com
Seeds, supplies, and information about sprouting.

Krispin Sullivan, C.N.
Clinical Nutrition
P.O. Box 961
Woodacre, CA 94973-0961
Phone: 415-488-9636
www.krispin.com or www.sunlightandvitamind.com
Clinical nutritionist; medical protocols for testing and treating vitamin D deficiencies.

Teldon of Canada, Ltd.
7432 Fraser Park Drive
Burnaby, BC V5J 5B9, Canada
Phone: 1-800-663-2212 or 604-436-0545
Fax: 604-435-4862
Home kefir makers with reusable kefir grains.

Weston A. Price Foundation
PMB 106-380
4200 Wisconsin Avenue, N.W.
Washington, DC 20016
Phone: 202-333-HEAL
www.westonaprice.org

NUTRITIONAL SUPPLEMENTS

Alternatives newsletter
Mountain Home Publishing
1201 Seven Locks Road
Rockville, MD 20854

Phone: 1-800-219-8591
www.drdavidwilliams.com
Monthly newsletter by David G. Williams, M.D.

Bio-Nutritional Formulas
106 East Jericho Turnpike
P.O. Box 311
Mineola, NY 11501-0311
Phone: 1-800-950-8484
Fax: 1-800-321-2573
Supplements, including thymic protein.

Golden Health Products, Inc.
6 Kentucky Road
Quincy, IL 62301
Phone: 1-800-780-1198
Seacure and other supplements.

Health Alert **newsletter**
5 Harris Court, N6
Monterey, CA 93940-5753
Phone: 831-372-2103
Monthly newsletter by Bruce West, D.C.

Healing Within Products, Inc.
84 Berkeley Avenue
San Anselmo, CA 94960
Phone: 1-800-30-7548 or 415-454-6677
Fax: 415-454-6659
Supplements, informative catalog.

Immune Systems Products
5 Harris Court, N6
Monterey, CA 93940
Phone: 1-800-231-8063 or 831-372-3805
Standard Process supplements, publishes product list with descriptions and recommendations.

Life Enhancement Products, Inc.
266 Saginaw Road
Sanford, MI 48657
Phone: 1-800-914-6311
Seacure and other supplements.

Life Enhancement Products, Inc.
P.O. Box 751390
Petaluma, CA 94975-1390
Phone: 1-800-543-3873 or 707-762-6144
Fax: 707-769-8016
www.life-enhancement.com
Dr. Jonathan Wright's Thyroplex thyroid supplement and other products.

Naturally Vitamins
14851 North Scottsdale Road
Scottsdale, AZ 85254
Phone: 1-800-899-4499
www.naturallyvitamins.com
Imports Wobenzym N from Germany, recommended for systemic oral enzyme therapy.

Nutrition Coalition
  P.O. Box 8023
  Fargo, ND 58109-8023
  Phone: 1-800-447-4793 or 701-235-4064
  Willard Water extract, colostrum supplements.

Nutrition and Healing **newsletter**
  Agora, Inc.
  819 N. Charles Street
  Baltimore, MD 21201
  Phone: 410-223-2611
  Monthly newsletter from Jonathan Wright, M.D.

Preventive Therapies, Inc.
  P.O. Box 956248
  Duluth, GA 30096
  Phone: 1-800-556-5530 or 770-409-0900
  Thymic supplement.

Rainbow Light Nutritional Systems
  125 McPherson Street
  Santa Cruz, CA 95060
  Advanced Enzyme System supplement for use with
  meals or between meals for systemic oral enzyme therapy.
  Sold in health food stores.

Standard Process, Inc.
1200 West Royal Lee Drive
Palmyra, WI 53156
Phone: 1-800-848-5061 or 414-495-2122
Fax: 414-495-2512
www.standardprocess.com
　　Product information available to licensed health care professionals, not retail customers. Vitamin, mineral, glandular, and food supplement products from organically grown whole-food sources. Available at some health food stores and mail-order suppliers, including Immune Systems Products (see separate listing).

The Vitamin Shoppe, Inc.
4700 Westside Avenue
North Bergen, NJ 07047
Phone: 1-800-223-1216 or 201-866-7711
Fax: 1-800-852-7153
　　Supplements by mail.

Willner Chemists
100 Park Avenue
New York, NY 10017
Phone: 1-800-633-1106 or 212-682-2817
Fax: 212-682-6192
　　Supplements by mail.

Wysong Institute
1880 North Eastman Road
Midland, MI 48642-7779
Phone: 517-631-0009
Fax: 517-631-8801
E-mail: wysong@tm.net
Food-source supplements.

MEDICINAL HERBS

American Botanical Council
P.O. Box 144345
Austin, TX 78714-4345
Phone: 512-926-4900
Fax: 512-926-2345
E-mail: abc@herbalgram.org or
custserve@herbalgram.org
www.herbalgram.org
Educational and research organization, publisher of
HerbalGram, quarterly magazine devoted to herbal medicine. Excellent resource.

American Herb Association
P.O. Box 1673
Nevada City, CA 95959
Educational organization, quarterly newsletter.

American Herbalists Guild
P.O. Box 746555
Arvada, CO 80006-6555
Phone: 303-423-8800
Fax: 303-428-8828
Professional organization, practitioners, referrals, quarterly newsletter.

The Herb Companion
Herb Companion Press
P.O. Box 55295
Boulder, CO 80322-5295
Phone: 1-800-456-5835
www.interweave.com
Bimonthly general interest magazine.

The Herb Quarterly
Long Mountain Press, Inc.
223 San Anselmo Avenue, Suite 7
San Anselmo, CA 94960
Quarterly general interest magazine.

HerbalGram
See American Botanical Council above.

Herb Pharm
P.O. Box 116
Williams, OR 97544
Phone: 1-800-348-4372 or 1-800-599-2392
Fax: 1-800-545-7392

Alkaloid-free comfrey tincture, arnica tincture, and other superior-quality herbs.

Herb Research Foundation
1007 Pearl Street, Suite 200
Boulder, CO 80302
Phone: 303-449-2265
Fax: 303-449-7849
E-mail: info@herbs.com
www.herbs.org
Library of 100,000 scientific articles on the safety and health benefits of herbs. Excellent resource.

Imhotep, Inc.
P.O. Box 183
Ruby, N.Y. 12475
Phone: 1-800-677-8577 or 845-336-2070
ProSeed grapefruit seed extract and related products.

International Herb Association
P.O. Box 317
Mundelein, IL 60060
Phone: 847-949-4372
Fax: 847-949-5896
E-mail: ihacathy@aol.com
Association of herb professionals. Newsletter, activities.

Jean's Greens
119 Sulphur Springs Road
Newport, NY 13416
Phone: 1-888-845-TEAS or 315-845-6500
Herbs, supplies, books, free reports on herbal topics.
Superior quality, inexpensive Essiac tea (brand name
Forticell).

Larreacorp, Ltd.
P.O. Box 6598
Chandler, AZ 85226
Phone: 1-800-682-9448
Fax: 602-963-7310
Larreastat chaparral extract, treated to remove potential
toxins.

Meadowbrook Herb Garden
93 Kingstown Road
Wyoming, RI 02898
Phone: 1-888-539-7603
Biodynamically grown (a step beyond organic) medic-
inal teas. Superior quality.

Northeast Herbal Association
P.O. Box 10
Newport, NY 13416
Educational, professional organization; journal, activities.

Nuherbs Co.
3820 Penniman Avenue
Oakland, CA 94619

Phone: 1-800-233-4307 or 510-534-4384
Fax: 1-800-550-1928 or 510-534-4384
Superior-quality Chinese herbs.

Nutri-Biotic
P.O. Box 238
Lakeport, CA 95453
Phone: 1-800-225-4345 *or* 707-263-0411
Fax: 707-263-7844
E-mail: nutribio@pacific.net
Grapefruit seed and related products.

Richters
357 Highway 47
Goodwood, Ontario, L0C 1A0 Canada
Phone: 905-640-6677
Fax: 905-640-6641
E-mail: orderdesk@richters.com
Outstanding free catalog of herb plants and seeds, excellent shipping service, superior quality; also sells dried herbs and books. With its photographs and concise descriptions of several hundred herbs, the catalog doubles as an herbal reference book.

Root to Health
P.O. Box 509
Wausau, WI 54402-0509
Phone: 1-800-388-3818 or 715-675-2326
Fax: 715-675-9730
E-mail: info@hsuginseng.com
Hsu's Ginseng. Excellent quality, informative catalog.

Sage Mountain Herb Products
P.O. Box 420
East Barre, VT 05649
Phone: 802-479-9825
Rosemary Gladstar's herbal products company.
Recommended.

Simplers Botanicals
P.O. Box 39
Forestville, CA 95436
Phone: 707-887-2012
Fax: 707-887-8570
James Green's herbal products company. Recommended.

United Plant Savers
P.O. Box 420
East Barre, VT 05649
Phone: 802-479-9825
Fax: 802-476-3722
E-mail: ups@ilhawaii.net
Nonprofit, grassroots organization for the restoration and cultivation of environmentally threatened medicinal plants.

AROMATHERAPY

Acqua Vita
85 Arundel Avenue
Toronto, Ontario, Canada M4K 3A3
Phone: 416-405-8855
E-mail: acquavita@interlog.com

Hydrosols therapeutic wall chart showing the known and experimental properties of forty aromatic distillates (hydrosols) and their applications. Therapeutic-quality hydrosols and essential oils from Suzanne Catty.

Aromaleigh, Inc.
180 St. Paul Street, #402
Rochester, NY 14604
Phone: 1-877-894-2283
www.aromaleigh.com
Aromatherapy products for pets and people from Kristen Leigh Bell.

Aromatic Plant Project
219 Carl Street
San Francisco, CA 94117
Phone: 415-564-5785
Fax: 415-564-5799
www.aromaticplantproject.com
Promotes the production and use of therapeutic-quality hydrosols and essential oils—products, projects, and newsletter.

Aromatic Thymes
P.O. Box 5041
Brentwood, TN 37024
Phone: 847-304-0975
Fax: 847-304-0989
www.aromaticthymes.com
Quarterly aromatherapy magazine.

JPT Aromatherapy
1901 Brule Street
South Lake Tahoe, CA 96150
Phone: 1-888-278-7364 or 530-577-5338
Fax: 530-577-5722
E-mail: jptaroma@thetahoe.net
The world's largest line of authentic wild and organic essential oils, including fifty hydrosols (true floral waters).

DETOXIFICATION

Golden Health Products, Inc.
6 Kentucky Road
Quincy, IL 62301
Phone: 1-800-780-1198
Seacure and other supplements.

Healing Within Products, Inc.
84 Berkeley Avenue
San Anselmo, CA 94960
Phone: 1-800-300-7548 or 415-454-6677
Fax: 415-454-6659
Citrus pectin, medicinal mushrooms, and other products that support detoxification.

The Heritage Store
P.O. Box 444
Virginia Beach, VA 23458-0444
Phone: 1-800-862-2923
Fax: 1-800-329-2292
Castor oil pack materials.

Immune System Products
5 Harris Court N6
Monterey, CA 93940
Phone: 1-800-231-8063 or 831-372-3805
  Natural, food-source supplements from Standard Process.

Jean's Greens
119 Sulphur Springs Road
Newport, NY 13416
Phone: 1-888-845-TEAS or 315-845-6500
  Essiac tea (brand name Forticell) and other herbs for detoxification.

Life Enhancement Products, Inc.
266 Saginaw Road
Sanford, MI 48657
Phone: 1-800-914-6311
  Seacure and other supplements.

Mayway Corporation
1338 Mandela Parkway
Oakland, CA 94607
Phone: 1-800-2-MAYWAY or 510-208-3113
Fax: 1-800-909-2828
E-mail: sales@mayway.com
  Minor Bupleurum Formula (Xiao Chai Hu Tang Wan) and other Chinese formulas.

Norimoor Company, Inc.
La Maison Francaise #5222
Fifth Avenue
New York, NY 10185-0043
Phone: 212-695-MOOR or 212-268-5399
Fax: 212-695-4535
Herbal Melange from Australia.

Nutrition Coalition
P.O. Box 8023
Fargo, ND 58109-8023
Phone: 1-800-447-4793 or 701-235-4064
Willard Water extract, colostrum supplements.

Pines International, Inc.
P.O. Box 1107
Lawrence, KS 66044-8107
Phone: 1-800-697-4637 or 913-841-6016
Fax: 913-841-1252
Superior-quality wheat grass and other grass powders and tablets.

Wysong Institute
1880 North Eastman Road
Midland MI 48642-7779
Phone: 517-631-0009
Fax: 517-631-8801
E-mail: wysong@tm.net
Natural, food-source supplements.

TREATING DIGESTIVE DISORDERS, ARTHRITIS, RHEUMATISM, JOINT PAIN, BREATHING DISORDERS, AND OTHER ACHES AND PAINS

Alive, **Canadian Journal of Health & Nutrition**
7436 Fraser Park Drive
Burnaby, BC V5J 5B9
Phone: 604-435-1919
Fax: 604-435-4888
Leading natural health magazine.

Alternative Medicine
P.O. Box 1056
Escondido, CA 92033-9871
Phone: 1-800-333-HEAL
www.alternativemedicine.com
Excellent bimonthly magazine.

Avena Botanicals
219 Mill Street
Rockport, ME 04856
Phone: 207-236-2121
Deb Soule's herbal apothecary; mail-order catalog.

B & B Marketing
569-B Holcombe Avenue
Mobile, AL 36606
Phone: 1-800-737-9295 or 334-476-9838
Fax: 334-476-7969
E-mail: Squillions@aol.com
Manufactures the Sacro Wedgy, a device that helps position the sacroiliac to relieve sciatica and back pain.

Sam Biser
Save Your Life Videos
P.O. Box 8122
Van Nuys, CA 91409-8122
Phone 1-800-926-4561 or 818-503-5980
Publishes *The Last Chance Health Report*, edited by Sam Biser. Back issues, including the 1993 report "Bone Regeneration: How to Regrow Damaged Kneecaps, Fractured Bones, and Repair Spinal Damage."

The Heritage Store
P.O. Box 444
Virginia Beach, VA 23458-0444
Phone: 1-800-862-2923
Fax: 1-800-329-2292
Edgar Cayce products, including herbs and castor oil pack materials.

Harmony Catalog
Gaiam, Inc.
360 Interlocken Boulevard, Suite 300
Broomfield, CO 80021

Phone: 1-800-869-3446
Fax: 1-800-456-1139
www.gaiam.com
Nontoxic products for house, garden, and personal use.
Ceramic Neti pot and HydroFloss dental irrigator. Air filters, allergy care products.

Karadsheh's Spice Bazaar, Inc.
3052 North 16th Street
Phoenix, AZ 85016
Phone: 1-800-307-7423
Fax: 602-277-0809
www.spicebazaar.com
Mastic gum.

Let's Live
P.O. Box 54192
Boulder, CO 80322-4192
Phone: 1-800-333-9951
Fax: 303-661-1816
Monthly natural health magazine.

NATR Inc.
2806 Broadway, Suite #2
Eureka, CA 95501
Phone: 1-800-422-4716 or 707-442-4716
Native-American tree resin (pitch) and olive oil ointments containing pitch. Pitch is a natural preservative and disinfectant.

Natural Health
70 Lincoln Street, 5th Floor
Boston, MA 02111
Phone: 617-753-8900
Fax: 617-457-0966
www.naturalhealthmag.com
Excellent monthly magazine.

Norimoor Company, Inc.
La Maison Francaise #5222,
Fifth Avenue
New York, NY 10185-0043
Phone: 212-695-MOOR or 212-268-5399
Fax: 212-695-4535
Herbal Melange from Austria.

Pines International, Inc.
P.O. Box 1107
Lawrence, KS 66044-8107
Phone: 1-800-697-4637 or 913-841-6016
Fax: 913-841-1252
Superior quality wheat grass and other grass powders
and tablets.

Therapeutic Botanicals, Inc.
2711 NW Sixth Street, Suite B
Gainsville, FL 32609
Phone: 1-877-890-6336 or 352-381-9496
Fax: 352-375-2663
    Organic neem products.

Wally's Natural Products
P.O. Box 5275
Auburn, CA 95604
www.wallysnatural.com
    Ear candles.

Index

('b' indicates boxed material)